T0173665

Using Voice and Theatre in Therapy

by the same author

Therapeutic Voicework
Principles and Practice for the Use of Singing as Therapy
Paul Newham
ISBN 1 85302 361 2

Using Voice and Movement in Therapy
The Practical Application of Voice Movement Therapy
Paul Newham
ISBN 1 85302 592 5

Using Voice and Song in Therapy
The Practical Application of Voice Movement Therapy
Paul Newham
ISBN 1 85302 590 9

of related interest

Sambadrama
The Arena of Brazilian Psychodrama
Edited and translated by Zoltán Figusch
Forewords by Adam Blatner and José Fonseca
ISBN 1 84310 363 X

Psychodrama
A Beginner's Guide
Zoran Djuri?, Jasna Veljkovi? and Miomir Tomi?
ISBN 1 84310 411 3

Rebels with a Cause
Working with Adolescents Using Action Techniques
Mario Cossa
Foreword by Zerka Moreno
ISBN 1 84310 379 6

Discovering the Self through Drama and Movement
The Sesame Approach
Edited by Jenny Pearson
ISBN 1 85302 384 1

Movement and Drama in Therapy, Second Edition
Audrey Wethered
ISBN 1 85302 199 7

Authentic Movement
Essays by Mary Starks Whitehouse, Janet Adler and Joan Chodorow
Edited by Patrizia Pallaro
ISBN 1 85302 653 0

Using Voice and Theatre in Therapy
The Practical Application of Voice Movement Therapy

Paul Newham

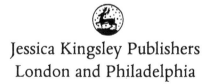

Jessica Kingsley Publishers
London and Philadelphia

First published in the United Kingdom in 2000
by Jessica Kingsley Publishers
116 Pentonville Road
London N1 9JB, UK
and
400 Market Street, Suite 400
Philadelphia, PA 19106, USA

www.jkp.com

Copyright © Paul Newham 2000
Printed digitally since 2006

The right of Paul Newham to be identified as author of this work has been
asserted by him in accordance with the Copyright, Designs and Patents Act
1988.

All rights reserved. No part of this publication may be reproduced in any
material form (including photocopying or storing it in any medium by
electronic means and whether or not transiently or incidentally to some other
use of this publication) without the written permission of the copyright owner
except in accordance with the provisions of the Copyright, Designs and Patents
Act 1988 or under the terms of a licence issued by the Copyright Licensing
Agency Ltd, 90 Tottenham Court Road, London, England W1T 4LP.
Applications for the copyright owner's written permission to reproduce any part
of this publication should be addressed to the publisher.

Warning: The doing of an unauthorised act in relation to a copyright work may
result in both a civil claim for damages and criminal prosecution.

Library of Congress Cataloging in Publication Data
A CIP catalog record for this book is available from the Library of Congress

British Library Cataloguing in Publication Data
A CIP catalogue record for this book is available from the British Library

ISBN-13: 978 1 85302 591 4
ISBN-10: 1 85302 591 7

Contents

Acknowledgements

I would like to acknowledge my appreciation to the following people. Dorothy Rosser for drawing Figures 4.11–4.18. Philip Grey for photographing and Alan Robertson for printing Figures 4.1 and 4.2. Helen Baggett for photographing and printing Figures 4.3–4.6. Nick Hale for photographing and printing Figures 4.7–4.10. I would also like to thank Jessica Kingsley Publishers for their commitment to the series of books of which this volume is a part.

Dedication

This book is dedicated to my dear friend and mentor Anne Kilcoyne whose ability to hear the psychological nuances of psyche's voice is unsurpassed. I thank her for hearing my voice in cacophony and melody, for directing my thoughts, and for choreographing my intuitions.

In her I found a model, a guide and a navigator.

Many a swaying vessel has she steered to earth.

Voice Movement Therapy
Towards an Integrated Model
of Expressive Arts Therapy

Over the past 15 years I have been developing a systematic methodology for using singing and vocalisation as a therapeutic modality. On a personal level, I think the genesis of my work originates in the acoustic cacophony of my childhood, where the angry vocal yells of my father and the sorrowful vocal cries of my mother provided the musical accompaniment to my days. On a professional level, my investigative work began with my search for a way of developing liberated vocal self-expression in people with severe mental and physical handicaps who could not speak but who produced a broad spectrum of non-verbal sounds.

Alone and without a model for what I was attempting to do, I spent many years crawling along the floor, gurgling, screeching, singing and mirroring the many sounds which my clients made in order that I might enter into their language rather than seeking to demand that they speak mine.

I found that with patience and an experimental spirit I could release a certain amount of muscular tension and facilitate a more liberated use of the voice in people whose verbal proficiency was limited or non-existent. With this vocal release my clients seemed also to access a certain positive emotional expression and an attitude of celebration, as though a certain anguish had been assuaged. The question then was what to do with these voices which emerged.

Simultaneous with my investigations into voice with handicapped people, I was working as a composer and vocalist, drawing inspiration and influence from a multicultural musical perspective. As my knowledge of the world's music broadened I began to hear parallels between certain vocal qualities in indigenous singing styles, particularly those of the East and Middle East, and the sounds made by my handicapped clients. Taking short frozen moments from a variety of singing styles and comparing them with short recordings of handicapped voices, I realised that it was often not possible to tell which was which. I then began to produce performances with my clients which choreographed their movements and orchestrated their vocal sounds to create impressionistic theatre pieces.

By combining my artistic research with a study of physiology, I began to evolve a method for using singing as a mode of artistic expression and therapeutic investigation with non-verbal populations. But the key to my work was the use of my own voice as a probe and a mirror. I learned to radically expand the tonal range and timbral malleability of my voice and use this instrument to communicate with my non-speaking clients. Though we could not speak with one another, we could sing – taking singing in its broadest sense. As my work expanded I was increasingly asked to train other professionals to make use of my methods and I gradually began to withdraw from working directly with handicapped people and started to work with professional care assistants, speech therapists, psychologists and a broad range of workers in the field of special education.

Because the exploration of my own voice had been so central to my investigations, my work with these new so-called 'able' clients took a very practical form. I offered one-to-one voice and singing lessons where the objective was not to produce a beautiful voice but to explore the complete vocal range, valuing all sounds as an authentic expression of the person. However, whereas the main obstacles to liberated vocal expression amongst my original handicapped clients had been neuromuscular, it seemed that my new clientele were inhibited and constricted primarily by psychological issues which manifested in various muscular tensions that inhibited and impeded liberated use of the voice. In addition, when I was able to facilitate vocal liberation, new-found sounds were often accompanied by intense emotions which in turn produced new sounds as my clients experienced a spectrum of feelings from deep grief to tumultuous joy, expressed through vocal qualities ranging from guttural bass to piercing soprano. I therefore realised that to progress with the development of my work, I had to understand thoroughly not only the physiological nature of vocal expression but also the relationship between voice and psyche. Consequently, I combined a theoretical study of physiology and psychotherapy with the undergoing of my own personal psychoanalysis.

In order to understand in more detail the physiological process of vocalisation I needed to observe the internal workings of my larynx whilst vocalising. I was therefore honoured and grateful when David Garfield-

Davies, at that time consultant laryngologist at the Middlesex Hospital, London, offered to make a video stroboscopic recording of my working larynx by threading a fibre optic camera through my nasal passages. This confirmed that the techniques I was forging not only enabled the vocal instrument to radically increase tonal range and timbral malleability, but they did so in a way entirely synonymous with healthy methods of voice production. Film of this can be seen on the accompanying video to this book, *Shouting for Jericho: The Work of Paul Newham on the Human Voice* (Newham 1997a). Meanwhile, I began to realise that many of the tenets of psychotherapy could be transposed from a verbal to a vocal mode of expression. I believed that I was establishing the idea of singing as therapy.

In time my one-to-one practice grew to include many other kinds of clients besides those who wanted to learn the principles of my work in order to apply it professionally. As my private practice of one-to-one voice sessions grew, I had the opportunity to apply my evolving systematic methodology of vocal work to a broad range of clients, some of whom came in the hope of alleviating physical problems such as constriction, asthma, and stammering, whilst others came for psychological reasons such as shyness, debilitating grief or repressed anger. The systematic approach which I had forged from my work with mentally and physically handicapped people was equally effective with this clientele and the added dimension of acknowledging the psychological significance of the process deepened the work with all clients.

Though each client brought with them into my consulting room unique issues which were worked through and explored not through speaking but through singing, I began to recognise certain approaches, exercises, methods and exploratory investigations which seemed to facilitate authentic vocal expression in all clients, regardless of their unique disposition.

Combining the use of my emerging system of vocal release with a unique personal psychotherapeutic relationship with each individual client I realised that I was creating the foundations for a therapeutic modality which compared to the expressive arts therapies – such as drama therapy and dance therapy – except where the channel of expression was voice and movement. I called this modality Voice Movement Therapy.

At the heart of my work was – and is – a systematic methodology for interpreting vocal sound. This system distills the voice into ten acoustic ingredients which emanate from physiological functioning, which provide a language for describing the voice and which relate to psychological, emotional and artistic expression. This system is described in detail in my book *Therapeutic Voicework: Principles and Practice for the Use of Singing as a Therapy* (Newham 1997b) and is presented in Chapter 3 of this volume. A concise recap of the system is also outlined briefly in Appendix 1 of this volume. Because of the difficulty inherent in attempting to describe vocal sounds in written words, I have published a set of audio cassette tapes *The Singing Cure: Liberating Self Expression Through Voice Movement Therapy* (Newham 1998) which explain the Voice Movement Therapy System of Vocal Analysis giving ample vocal examples of the spectrum of vocal sounds in speech and song which arise from different combinations of the ten core ingredients. Details of how to obtain accompanying resources to this book and access other information regarding Voice Movement Therapy is given in Appendix 2 of this volume.

Before long, I had more clients and more work than I could possibly handle. I therefore considered that I could actually reach more clients by training others to impart the work as facilitators, voice coaches, singing teachers, therapists, special education workers and community leaders; so I began running short courses in the techniques and methodologies which I had forged.

In the summer following the first series of short courses, I became unable to work due to exhaustion, and a graduate of one of my training courses, Jenni Roditi, offered to take over my client practice. In doing this, Roditi verified that the techniques were indeed grounded and practicable enough to be passed on and administered by others with equal efficacy as when administered by myself.

On returning to teaching the courses which I was developing, and as I observed graduates apply the work in various settings, I began to be convinced that there was a need for more trained and qualified practitioners who could use voice to facilitate a therapeutic process which yielded liberated self-expression in others. I therefore developed the short courses which I had been teaching into a full professional training leading to a professional Diploma in Voice Movement Therapy, which is currently accredited by the Oxford and Cambridge University and Royal Society of Arts Examinations Board. The major focus of my work is now directing this professional training in Voice Movement Therapy and teaching other short courses in specific areas of the work.

The professional training course in Voice Movement Therapy provides a thorough practical, experiential and technical education in an approach to working therapeutically with the voice which synthesises the physiological, artistic, psychological and educational aspects of vocal work in a single strategy. Because of its broad but integrated nature, it has attracted students from many backgrounds from all over the world. Trainees include musicians or performing artists seeking to develop their vocal and compositional skills; psychotherapists seeking to incorporate vocal work into their approach; speech and language therapists seeking an integrated and experiential model to complement their allopathic training; freelance peripatetic group leaders who run workshops and offer sessional work for a variety of client groups; and many others whose professional intention is unclear but who seek a personal vocational training which unites exploration of the Self with the acquisition of technical skills. The diverse student fraternity provides a particularly fertile environment and graduates utilise the work in very different ways. Some graduates work with clients or patients in clinical institutions or in one-to-one practice; some devise performances and lead experiential workshops; some offer vocal training in drama schools and in individual client practice; some combine the vocal work with other arts therapies or with physical therapies; and others work in a way that combines a number of different models.

Although the designing and teaching of this course in many ways provided a culmination to my intentions, there was still a missing link. For, on graduating from the training course, practitioners encounter many complex issues relating to the practice of Voice Movement Therapy for which they need further support, supervision, guidance and a sense of being part of a network. I therefore formed the International Association for Voice Movement Therapy which is governed by a code of ethics and a constitution and to which qualified graduate practitioners of Voice Movement Therapy belong. This Association is in its early days but provides an entirely necessary forum for the supervision of practitioners and an investigation of issues relating to the practice of a therapeutic approach to vocal expression.

In seeking to ground Voice Movement Therapy practically and theoretically, I have been driven to thoroughly research the cross-cultural evolution of a therapeutic approach to vocal expression from ancient shamanic practices and spiritual healing to avant-garde theatre and present-day psychotherapy; and my research has uncovered a rich history of investigation into the healing use of singing and non-verbal vocal expression in many areas and through many ages. This research has enabled me to develop a consolidated body of vocal work which synthesises the practical application of principles drawn from a range of disciplines including psychotherapy, massage, remedial voice training, stress management, singing, music, ethnomusicology and special needs education. The discovery of other previous approaches enabled me to understand what I was doing as the synthesising of fragments emanating from an existing tradition.

Being sceptical of anything which claims to be new and having a deep respect for tradition, I felt determined to ensure that I brought the long-standing practice of a therapeutic approach to vocal expression to the attention of present-day practitioners and students within the relevant professions. I was therefore honoured when Jessica Kingsley invited me to publish a complete and unabridged history of the use of voice and singing in therapy. In that book, *Therapeutic Voicework: Principles and Practice for the Use of Singing as a Therapy* (Newham 1997b), I have described the theoretical and practical history of the subject. In addition, throughout *Therapeutic Voicework* I have related the various historic and extant approaches to vocal expression to the techniques of Voice Movement Therapy. However, the description of practical techniques and theoretical principles relating specifically to the dramatic and theatrical nature of vocal expression is a small part of what is primarily a historical and theoretical overview of the entire field.

In this book, *Using Voice and Theatre in Therapy: The Practical Application of Voice Movement Therapy*, I intend to focus specifically on the area of drama and theatre, investigating the way that the therapeutic application of vocal expression can be informed by an appreciation of twentieth-century European theatre processes. This book is the third in a series of three volumes which concern the practical application of Voice Movement Therapy. These books are a description of Voice Movement Therapy for those interested in the nitty gritty of using voice and movement as a therapeutic tool. For it has come to my attention over the past few years that there is an ever increasing interest in the therapeutic value of singing and non-verbal vocal expression amongst therapists from all orientations. Such professionals and students of the therapies are often eager to have an insight into how a therapeutic modality with singing and voice at its centre actually works in practice. In this book I shall seek to throw some light on this enquiry and I hope that those seeking to acquaint themselves with an integrated and coherent model of therapeutic vocal work may find inspiration, information and affirmation. Readers interested in a complete historic and theoretical background to the therapeutic use of vocal expression are referred to my earlier book *Therapeutic Voicework* (Newham 1997b).

Most therapists, teachers and other practitioners working with the hearts and souls of other people recognise that the human voice is a primary medium of communication in human beings. It is an expression of who we are and how we feel. In the timbre of a person's voice you can hear the subtle music of feeling and thought. The ever shifting collage of emotions which we experience infiltrate the voice with tones of happiness, excitement, depression and grief. The human voice is also one way in which we preserve our identity; and the voice and the psychological state of an individual mutually influence each other. The physical condition of the body is also reflected in the vitality of vocal expression: illness, physical debilitation and habitual muscular patterns all take their toll on the way we sound. The voice is both an expression of psychological state, a physiological operation and the means by which a person asserts his or her rights within the social order. But many people find themselves negatively affected by psychological dynamics such as stress, anxiety and depression, by physical factors resulting from congenital conditions, illness, injury or bodily misuse and by socially enforced inhibitions. If these effects continue unabated, they often begin to reduce the agility and vitality of body and voice and thereby deplete the capacity for unencumbered expression.

Because the voice is composed of such a complex set of dimensions, the condition of vocal inhibition, restraint or depleted function, from which so many people suffer, leads to an expressive impairment on a psychological, physiological and social level. To reverse the process and revive vocal function therefore necessitates attention to both psychological, physical and social processes. Providing these processes are properly understood, working with the voice can be an enlivening way of helping people overcome difficulties which hinder the acoustic and kinetic expression of the Self. And such work may be called Voicework.

Voicework may perhaps best be described as a generic term which includes any work with or on the voice. Within this definition a singing teacher could be said to practise Voicework in developing the vocal skills of her pupils; a bereavement counsellor could be said to practise Voicework in helping a client feel safe and comfortable in giving voice to grief; a speech and language therapist conducts Voicework in helping a patient be relieved of pathological conditions which threaten the health of the voice; a choir leader may be said to practise Voicework in enabling a mass of disparate voices to synthesise into a harmonious whole; a gestalt psychotherapist may draw upon Voicework in assisting a client to give vent to rage through shouts and yells; a *répétiteur* conducts Voicework when she helps an anxious opera singer with the task of sustaining the demands of the music whilst articulating the poetic text; a music therapist uses Voicework when she helps a young child create a song from a simple rhyme; a priest employs Voicework when using the tonal contours of his voice to communicate to the congregation; a politician uses Voicework when he deliberately employs specific vocal timbres to convince and persuade.

All of these people are using the voice as a channel through which to express or 'push out' something from the inside; and the voice is indeed a major bridge between the inner world of mood, emotion, image, thought and experience and the outer world of relationship, discourse and interaction.

Because the voice is so intimately connected to the expression of feelings and ideas and is a primary channel through which we communicate who we are, Voicework is often innately therapeutic. However, the term Voicework is not synonymous with 'voice therapy'.

The term 'voice therapy' denotes a clinical allopathic field of work conducted by 'voice therapists' who are speech and language therapists with a specialisation in voice disorders. It is also true, however, that a number of medical doctors who have specialised in ear, nose and throat dysfunction and disease (ENT) and who have a special focus on laryngological problems may also call themselves voice therapists. Both ENT doctors and speech therapists alleviate a wide range of disorders and, though both kinds of practitioners approach the voice as a somatic phenomenon, increasing numbers of doctors as well as speech and language therapists are beginning to incorporate attendance to the influence of emotional and psychological factors upon the voice.

Although strictly speaking the term 'voice therapy' designates the aforementioned field, in recent years an increasing number of people working in the broad area of 'complementary', 'alternative' or 'holistic' medicine have utilised the term 'voice therapy' to denote the process by which vocalisation through speech, song and non-verbal sound is used as a means through which to express and explore aspects of the psyche. These practitioners utilise the term 'therapy' for its psychic rather than its somatic implication, inviting comparison with the work of psychotherapists rather than speech and language therapists or ENT consultants. However, few of these practitioners are trained in psychotherapy or counselling; which adds further confusion to the vernacular meaning and signification of the term 'voice therapy'. There are also many artistic practitioners, some of long-standing excellence, particularly within the field of the avant-garde experimental theatre, who describe their teaching as being, in part, a therapy. This invites the work of theatre practitioners who impart or facilitate vocal work, such as directors, actors and workshop leaders, to be compared to that of a drama therapist. Yet few of these artists are drama therapists. There are also many individuals working in community centres with so-called handicapped children, in mental health wings of hospitals, in special schools and in the voluntary sector who are 'helping' others towards positive change and thus are working therapeutically. Those who utilise vocal expression as part of their approach may understandably be perceived as disseminating 'voice therapy'; yet few of these people have a therapeutic training or qualification.

The widespread use of the term 'therapy' in general and 'voice therapy' specifically is therefore beginning to denote a broad style of work and a particular kind of outcome rather than identifying someone who is trained and qualified in a therapeutic discipline. Furthermore, the word 'therapy', particularly in the current political climate, is subject to so much scrutiny and currently designates such a broad field that it is, for many, time to consider carefully the variety of meanings which the term has.

My assertion is that all approaches to Voicework can most certainly be therapeutic. Moreover, its therapeutic effects can be somatic as well as psychological. This does not, however, necessarily mean that all Voicework practitioners are therapists or that all approaches to Voicework are therapeutic. In fact, many people have suffered the most abominable anti-therapeutic treatment in the hands of voice coaches, singing teachers and voice workshop leaders who, whilst artistically and technically competent in the field of voice, have not the slightest insight into the foundations of compassion and analysis upon which a truly therapeutic contract is built.

Voice Movement Therapy may be described as a particular approach to Voicework and a specifically crafted form of therapeutic Voicework. Voice Movement Therapy can help people whose expressive activity has been detrimentally influenced by emotional problems, trauma and mental illness, those whose lives have been turned around by the effects of severe injury or the development of diseases such as Multiple Sclerosis, those with congenital conditions such as Cerebral Palsy and Down's Syndrome and those who have been discouraged from asserting or expressing themselves by overpowering and infertile environmental influences. In addition, Voice

Movement Therapy can respond to the needs of those whose social or professional predicament places exceptional demands upon the voice, who often find themselves ill-equipped to preserve the health and longevity of their vocal instrument and therefore require education and rehabilitation. No less important are those who, whilst healthy and not overtly impeded, can nonetheless discover an increased potential for expression and creativity through singing and sound-making.

If not conducted with skill and expertise, however, Voice Movement Therapy can also be threatening to the health of mind and body; and there are some people for whom any kind of therapeutic Voicework, including Voice Movement Therapy, may not be expedient to the maintenance of health no matter how proficient the practitioner. Consequently, someone practising any kind of Voicework needs to be competent in understanding the psychophysical nature of vocal expression; and in addition must learn to recognise those for whom Voicework is an inappropriate medium through which to work for physical or psychological reasons.

In my view, though there are many resourceful, sensitive and proficient voice practitioners administering many diverse approaches to Voicework, some therapeutic and some not, any Voicework practitioner, particularly a practitioner working with an overt therapeutic dimension, should be trained to do so.

All students of the professional training in Voice Movement Therapy undergo a thorough physical and psychological journey in order to facilitate the same in others. In addition, all trainees study creative, allopathic and psychological models of intervention and analysis. They are thereby trained to be practitioners who can deal effectively with the psychological and physical aspects of vocal expression and who, in suspecting serious pathology of mind or body, will refer the client to an appropriate practitioner.

Voice Movement Therapy can be conducted with individuals and with groups. The clients begin by making their most effortless natural sound whilst the acoustic tones of the voice and the muscle tone of the body are heard and observed. In response to an informed analysis of breathing, sound and movement the practitioner massages and manipulates the client's body, gives instruction in ways of moving and suggests moods and images which the client allows to affect and infiltrate the vocal timbre. The voice is thereby sculptured and animated through a graphic and authentic expression of the Self. In order to facilitate this process, the practitioner also offers pedagogic technical training by which the voice develops in range and malleability; this helps the client find access to sounds which give expression to hitherto dormant aspects of the Self. The result of such Voicework is psychologically uplifting, physically invigorating, creatively rejuvenating and serves to release vocal function from constriction.

As the process unfolds, the client is encouraged and enabled to use creative writing from which lyrics for songs are drawn. The practitioner then helps the client create songs which are vocalised using the broadest possible range of the voice, giving artistic expression to personal material. In addition, the spectrum of voices which are elicited during the process are also used as the basis from which to create characters which symbolise and express different aspects of the Self. Voice Movement Therapy thereby draws on dance, music and drama and in many ways, therefore, provides a model for an integrated expressive arts therapy where creative movement, creative writing, music and theatre are synthesised into a coherent strategy within which all strands are linked by the common thread of the voice. However, Voice Movement Therapy differs from other arts therapies in that it necessarily appropriates a physiological dimension, as the voice is so often the locus for somatic and psychosomatic difficulties – and a complete understanding of vocal expression is not possible without an appreciation of the way the voice functions physiologically.

The techniques which constitute Voice Movement Therapy can, therefore, be loosely divided into three areas. The first of these areas is the use of voice with movement, dance and massage and is covered in the first volume of this series: *Using Voice and Movement in Therapy* (Newham 1999a). The second area is the use of voice with creative writing and singing, which is covered in Volume Two: *Using Voice and Song in Therapy* (Newham 1999b). The third area is the use of voice with drama and performance, which is covered in this volume: *Using Voice and Theatre in Therapy*.

These books aim to be both theoretically informative and practically inspiring. For, though the use of Voice Movement Therapy as a mode of therapeutic enquiry, like all disciplines, requires training, there are parts of the Voice Movement Therapy methodology which therapists from other orientations can borrow from, adapt and utilise. I hope that the techniques described in this book will inspire practitioners to broaden their field of enquiry to include vocal expression.

Naturally, the untrained, unconsidered use of vocal expression in a therapeutic context is potentially dangerous; and many of the techniques which constitute Voice Movement Therapy require practical training to know how to administer them. This is not a handbook. At the end of the day, each reader must employ discernment in keeping with the nature of the subject.

In this book I not only give case studies but also reprint clients' own accounts of their experience of the work; and I am grateful to those who have permitted me to tell their story and quote their words. Nonetheless, names and other details have been altered to preserve confidentiality and anonymity.

CHAPTER I

The Roots of Human Diversity
Voice and Psyche in Archetypal Psychology

The Psychology of Theatre

Theatre is a magical arena within which fantasy and reality, truth and pretence, actuality and illusion intersect and convene with an alchemical mystery. Yet often theatre is composed of the most simple, pedestrian and ordinary. Indeed our expressions become theatre the moment someone is watching.

The performer occupies a special place in all cultures – in some the performer executes the rituals which accompany birth and death. In other societies, the performer is a medicine man or woman, using song and dance to heal; in some places the performer is an idol to be worshipped; in others the performer is a teller of tales, personifying stories that would otherwise be lost. In some contexts the performer dons masks and costumes which give the appearance of a special being from another world. In other places, the actors must convince the audience of their ordinary reality. Yet despite the differences, all performers use the same tools: voice and movement. For an actor, the voice and the body are the channels used for communicating the inner world of mood, emotion, thought and image to an audience.

The art of the theatre gives creative shape to a rudimentary psychological reality. For we are each made up of many characters, playing each one as the moment requires. The idea that we can 'give voice' to different aspects of ourselves, just as the actor gives voice to different characters, is embedded in the foundations of twentieth-century psychology. Theatre is an essential therapeutic tool because the psyche may be said to behave according to a dramatic model. And central to this model is the human voice as an expression of psychological diversity.

Jung's Complex

In 1904 Jung conducted some remarkable experiments with words which led to the discovery of the 'complex'. Jung took a group of healthy adults and read to each one in turn a list of 400 words. After hearing each word the subject was asked to respond with the first word which came into his or her head; this response and the time it took was then recorded. Sometimes the responses to certain words were simple and predictable, for example to the word 'window' a volunteer would reply 'pane' and to the word 'house' the reply would be 'roof'. However, some of the responses seemed at first rather unusual, for example to the word 'window' the volunteer would say 'cat', and to the word 'house' the reply would be 'lost'. On closer examination of the person's personal circumstances it was revealed that certain words produced seemingly odd reactions because they were connected to a specific emotionally charged preoccupation which the subject had, but of which he or she was unaware. For example, the person may respond to the word 'house' with 'lost' because of having narrowly escaped a fire when a child in which the house was lost or destroyed by the blaze; in a similar connection, the reply of 'cat' to the word 'window' may originate in the memory of seeing the pet cat in the window of the blazing furnace. Because of the extreme emotions associated with such an event, words which denote aspects of the experience serve to reanimate a faint and unconscious memory of it, including the re-experiencing of the appropriate emotions in a mild form. This is what Jung named the 'complex', which he defined as a network or cluster of half-forgotten single images which are held together by an emotional tone, in this case terror, which, though a person is not aware of it, can continue to affect him or her for a long time.

In each person there are many complexes which arise and dissolve as part of the natural process of shifting preoccupations; it is from them that we draw our moods, our feelings and our reactions. However, because the complexes are unconscious we are often at a loss to know where these forces come from. Many of the complexes, arising as they do from traumatic circumstances, are too painful to be allowed to remain in our field of attention, but they sustain a certain dormant life of their own. When things or events around us stimulate the recollection of previous experiences and thereby provoke a memory of the emotion originally attached to that experience, the complex is then activated and we experience feelings and behave in ways which seem strange. Complexes then are not a disease, they are not a sign of disorder or disturbance, on the contrary, they are the very means by which we feel. As

Jung said, 'there is no one who has no complexes, just as there is no one who is without emotions' (Jung 1953, Volume 2).

Ego in the Middle

Though we have many complexes, there is one particular network of images which is, at least in the healthy individual, dominant and central and to which Jung referred as the 'ego'. Thus, although the complexes dance a tango upon the stage of the psyche, the ego is at work like an organising centre without which we would have no constant identity and consequently our changes of mood would make us feel like a completely different personality each time an emotional transition occurred.

The ego is not one thing but a complex of sense-impressions and images, networks of ideas which we associate with the 'feeling-tone' of our own body. For Jung, the ego is, to a large extent, a conglomeration of the information which we receive through sight, hearing, taste, touch and smell. It is by way of the ego's association with the body that 'I' feel bunged up when my body is bronchially congested, or that 'I' feel aggravated when my skin is irritated. Jung said 'one's own personality is therefore the firmest and strongest complex', and 'good health permitting' it 'weathers all psychological storms' because 'the ego-complex, by reason of its direct connection with bodily sensations, is the most stable and the richest in associations' (Jung 1953, Volume 3).

The ego is, however, influenced by the other complexes which constantly guide us in what we do; for even though they are unconscious they actively cause us to carry out certain modes of behaviour. This gives them the appearance of independent beings, acting of their own accord, which is why Jung described the complexes as 'little people', 'mini-personalities' and 'splinter psyches'. This autonomy is due to the affect, feeling-tone or emotion that binds them together. Emotion is such a strong influence compared to the reason of the ego that any group of images which are united by a strong affect will always have their way. The emotion of terror at our house being burnt down is much stronger than the reason which tells us it is all in the past, it is this very strength that causes us to bury it; but it lives on with its own independence. Jung said that because emotion 'occupies in the constitution of the psyche a very independent place' the complexes are 'relatively independent of the central control of the consciousness, and at any moment liable to bend or cross the intentions of the individual' (Jung 1953, Volume 2).

Sometimes, if there are two or more complexes at work at the same time, the ego may become confused, feeling pulled first this way and then that. In a healthy individual the ego is so strong that it can take account of these voices and have the final say. But if the ego becomes weakened it gets lost, becoming only one voice amongst many. In such cases the psyche splits up into a multitude of voices all clamouring for domination. This is precisely what happens in some kinds of psychoses where Jung says 'the psychic totality falls apart' and 'splits up into complexes' such that 'the ego-complex ceases to play the important role amongst these' but 'is now just one among several complexes which are all equally important, or perhaps even more important than the ego' (Jung 1953, Volume 3).

Because the ego is affirmed and maintained primarily through its association with the body, such a swallowing of the ego by the other complexes gives rise to a so-called 'mind–body split' where the body becomes the seat of sensations which come from the complexes rather than from the outside world. This is also what can happen in schizophrenia. If our subject who lost her house becomes schizophrenic, her body may genuinely feel burned when she touches a cat and she may refuse to touch any windows for fear of getting burnt. In these circumstances the voice of the fire-complex is stronger than that of the ego and to the outside world these imaginings are so illogical that we cannot hope to penetrate their meaning; the 'hot cat' remains an absurdity to us. This resulting experience of the domination or submersion of the ego by one or more of the complexes is called a 'dissociation of personality'.

It is not irrelevant that Jung referred to the emotional binding of the complex as a 'tone', which is a musical, acoustic and therefore a vocal phenomenon. For Jung himself was to observe the activity and expression of the complexes through the timbral and tonal quality of the human voice.

Dead Men Singing

For his medical thesis, Jung studied the extraordinary case of a fifteen and a half-year-old girl who acted as a medium for the voices of the dead. Jung attended her regular seances where he witnessed these dead people express themselves through the girl's voice. Each time the girl expressed a different character, the quality or timbre of her voice would completely change. On occasions this involved major transformations of dialect and accent from German to French or Italian. Furthermore, though the girl displayed only a faint knowledge of High German in her normal life, in her trance she spoke the language faultlessly (Jung 1953, Volume 1). Jung later understood that these characters were different aspects of the girl's own personality, ramifications of her autonomous complexes; for she was undergoing a dissociation of her personality and it was through her voice that the complexes took on an identity which could be communicated to those observing.

Later, Jung noticed how those who in his day were diagnosed as schizophrenics often talked to themselves in voices with very different qualities; and he noted that in severe cases of psychotic disturbance the words of the voices degenerated into a pure muddle with no linguistic meaning. For example, he observed a catatonic who used to sing a religious song 'for hours on end' with the refrain 'Hallelujah' which over a period of months 'gradually degenerated' into 'Hallo', then 'Oha', and finally simply 'ha-ha-ha' which was 'accompanied by convulsive laughter'. Jung concluded that in schizophrenia 'eventually all words can be replaced by a "hm-hm-hm"' which is 'uttered in a stereotyped manner'. What remained was the tone in both senses: the emotional tone of the complex which was expressed through the audible vocal tone of the voice. For the psychotic does not hear a jumbled semi-verbal word salad in monotone, but in pitches and timbral qualities expressive of the affect of the complex. One is aggressive, spiteful and provocative, the other luring, sly and seductive, another Italian, confident and full of bravado, the other English, polite and reserved. The voices of psychoses each have characteristics expressed vocally through an acoustic tone whether there are words present or not. Thus, in vocal terms we might describe the concept of 'tone' as the affective nucleus of a complex as expressed through the acoustic quality of the voice.

The degeneration of a word salad into a purely vocal composition which Jung observed in schizophrenia has a parallel in bodily movements. The psychotic patient will, in the early stages of the disorder, repeat movements which have their genesis in some domestic gestural act, such as smoking a cigarette or combing the hair. Eventually, however, these movements become more and more abstracted until it is impossible for a newcomer to recognise where they originated. Jung observed such a choreographic degeneration in a patient who 'used to comb his hair a few hours every day in a stereotyped manner' claiming that he was seeking to remove the 'plaster that had been rubbed into it during the night'. Then, as the years went on 'the comb got further and further away from his head' until after three years of this dance the patient 'beat and scratched his chest' with the comb (Jung 1953, Volume 3).

About Archetypes

Though the complexes are often formed as the result of personal memories, usually of a distressing nature, there are other networks of images which have not been formulated through experience but have been inherited as so-called instincts. These may be described as patterns of behaviour, ways of reacting to things that you can guarantee observing in all human beings. These instincts are readily observed in animals. For example, we may observe the inherited instincts in young chicks whom we know are killed and eaten by hawks but not by gulls. If you take a group of chicks and enclose them in a cage before they have had any contact with the world, and draw a stuffed gull along a wire above them, the chicks will not react. If you take a stuffed hawk and draw it backwards across the cage, they still will not react. But if you draw it forwards the chicks begin digging and scratching, cooing and clucking in an attempt to get away. In this tiny creature there is therefore an inherited instinct of fear and flight that is attached to a certain image both in form and motion. If such an animal can possess such complicated inherited information, imagine what human beings inherit.

These inherited instincts are like complexes in that they cause us to react in a certain way. They lie beneath the personal unconscious in a stratum of the psyche called the 'collective unconscious'. They are known as 'archetypes' and cause us to execute certain modes of behaviour at certain times. For example, in every person there lies a certain appetite or instinct for childlike mischief which may be expressed as a playful desire for frivolity or by playing devil's advocate in a conversation; it may manifest as an evil desire to mock or ridicule someone's success; it might cause us to contemplate stealing something for the sheer thrill of it; or to torment someone by hiding their belongings. At such times we might say that the Trickster Archetype is dominating our behaviour. However, Jung looked not only at the way these archetypes gain expression through the way people behave but also through the images contained in dreams, fairy tales, myths, legends, poetry and painting. In writing we see the Trickster Archetype reflected in characters such as Dickens' Artful Dodger from the novel *Oliver Twist* who dances quick-foot between the crowds, picking the pockets of the local gentry; in the fairy-tale character of Rumpelstiltskin who plays a wicked trick of mischief in posing the riddle of his name; in Puck of Shakespeare's *A*

Midsummer Night's Dream who pours love juice into the wrong eyes and causes the havoc of infatuation; in Eros of Greek mythology who causes people to fall into the mischief of love by infecting them with his poisonous arrows; or in Penguin from the Batman story who incessantly devises more mean tricks to outwit the hero. All cultures have their examples of the childlike mischiever, for it is a universal and primordial instinct, it is the archetype of the Trickster.

Another important archetype is the Mother, a central figure to the art, culture and mythology of all peoples and always characterised by certain qualities. The Mother is the great nourisher, nurturing our growth with the milk of human kindness, she provides warmth and comfort reminiscent of the womb; she is the protector and life-giver. However, all archetypes have a positive and a negative side. Just as the Trickster is not only the harmless pickpocket but also the wicked conniver, causing death in the trail of his traps, so too the Mother has a dark side. Just as we would all love a taste of that ultimate dependence upon the Mother reminiscent of the womb, so too we fear our independence being consumed by the Mother's arms, for part of the Mother's dark side is her inability to let her children go. She is the suffocater who swallows her children whole, thwarting their independence and thus their very life.

The representation of the archetypes often takes the form not of a character but of an object or an animal. The Trickster may appear as a magpie or a fox. The Mother, in her bright aspect, may appear as a safe haven, a cave where the evil men on our trail will not find us, or as a cool pool of water in which we swim, kept buoyant by the nourishing minerals. In her dark aspect the Mother may appear as the dragon that will swallow us up, or the great hole in the earth that we fall into just before we wake up with a jump. All these archetypes play themselves out through our behaviour at different times and thus Jung discovered two levels to the unconscious psyche, the first he called the 'personal unconscious' and the second the 'collective unconscious'. In the personal unconscious reside all the complexes of images grouped according to our personal experience; whilst the collective unconscious houses the patterns that we have inherited. Jung therefore defined the personal unconscious as 'the totality of all psychic phenomena that lack the quality of consciousness' including 'all lost memories', 'all contents that are still too weak to become conscious' and 'all more or less intentional repressions of painful thoughts and feelings'. Meanwhile, he defined the collective unconscious as a receptacle for those 'qualities that are not individually acquired but are inherited', such as the 'instincts as impulses to carry out actions from necessity, without conscious motivation'. In addition, the collective unconscious houses the 'archetypes of perception and apprehension'. For, 'just as his instincts compel man to a specifically human mode of existence, so the archetypes force his ways of perception and apprehension into specifically human patterns' (Jung 1953, Volume 8).

The constant appearance and influence of both the personal complexes and the collective archetypes led Jung to propose that each of us is not one, but many, and that we all have multiple voices which need to have their say. Jung believed that the original state of the psyche is 'one in which the psychic processes are very loosely knit and by no means form a self-orientated unity' (Jung 1953, Volume 8). Jung asserted that daily life consists of a continuous dialogue between the many voices of the psyche and that this dialogue is absolutely crucial to a healthy and balanced life. Only through 'hearing out' the different possibilities, needs, moods, complexes and archetypal influences that a person has can he or she appreciate what it is to be alive.

Dreaming in Tongues

In the schizophrenics of his day, Jung observed merely an exaggerated form of the dialogue, necessary for healthy living, between different voices in the psyche. But, whereas for most people this dialogue is chaired by the dominating strength of the ego, in schizophrenia and other forms of psychotic experience, each of the voices acquire such an increased intensity that the ego becomes swamped and the psyche becomes saturated with a chorus of voices, each wanting to instigate a different mode of behaviour. For the healthy person with a strongly affirmed ego, however, Jung proclaimed the importance of maintaining a dialogue between the many voices. To this end, Jung proclaimed that 'one should nurture the art of conversing with oneself' and openly encouraged people to develop the ability to give each of their complexes a voice (Jung 1953, Volume 7). Indeed for Jung, this was one of the primary roles of psychotherapy. Furthermore, for Jung, anything which enabled a balanced conversance and interplay between the different voices was in itself therapeutic. Jung was therefore keen to observe many processes which gave outward manifestation to the inner psychic voices including painting, poetry, drama, opera and above all dreaming.

Jung believed that the psyche retains many ideas, images and linguistic symbols which originate from humankind's earliest days, through a genealogical inheritance. For Jung, there is a vast spectrum of image-matrices comprising emotions, instincts, ideas and characters to which the human psyche or imagination plays host. For Jung, all the characters and narratives which formulate religious mythology reflect the structure of and thus provide an allegorical metaphor for internal psychological processes, as it is from them that they emanate.

Jung conducted extensive cross-references between individual dreams and fantasies observing how their structure was represented in different guises in every individual in every culture. He consequently revealed how the roots and significance of symptoms and dream-images originate not in the sociological circumstances which influence the development of individual consciousness, but in unconscious universal structures, a system of 'genetic blue prints' or archetypes, which are continually reinvented through the personages which appear in myths and are continually reanimated through the process of dreaming. Jung believed that in dreaming as in psychoses there are 'numberless interconnections to which one can find parallels only in mythological associations of ideas' or 'poetic creations' which have often been borrowed from myths. Instead of tracing the significance of a dream to the idiosyncratic stories of the patient's daily life, Jung traced them to the larger stories of the myths, to ascertain which archetypal pattern the dream originated in. Thus, for Jung there were 'not only typical dreams but typical motifs in the dreams' which may be 'situations or figures' (Jung 1953, Volume 9, Part 1). For Jung, words were less important than the analysis of the dream contents as a pictorial symbol. Language was but the necessary means by which analyst and patient communicate; a transcription of the actual material, which, for Jung, was always symbolic. For Jung, a dream of flying, for example, took place in the context of universal myths where flight symbolised freedom, spirituality, heavenly ascension, escape and a host of other significations. Jung's method of dream analysis amplified the patient's image of flight and looked at all the other motifs which often occur alongside flight in mythical stories and he was thereby able to relate the age-old wisdom contained in the relevant myths to the life predicament of the patient.

In tracing patients' dreams to myths, Jung consequently raised their attention above a preoccupation with their own problems and dilemmas and enabled them to see that they were not alone in their suffering, but that they were temporarily hosting the eternal problems of humanity. For Jung, the individual suffering revealed through the psychotherapeutic process 'is archetypal and collective' and can be 'taken as a sign' that 'none of us is suffering for himself, but rather from the spirit of the age', that is 'from an objective, impersonal cause' or most succinctly from a 'collective unconscious which' each of us has 'in common with all men' (Jung 1953, Volume 5). Jung therefore developed an ever deepening respect for the ability of ancient myth to offer a timeless, figurative and allegorical reflection of a person's inner psychic life.

About the Self

Jung's vision of men's and women's psychological functioning was one which perceived the psyche as essentially multiple, a matrix of individual images and voices, part personal, part archetypal, which 'do not form a self-orientated unity' (Jung 1953, Volume 7). Jung observed the most overt example of this disorientated mass of images and voices in the behavioural manifestations of the so-called psychotic, in whom the extreme degree of autonomy in the emotion or affect which cemented the various image-matrices led to the appearance of a number of separate personalities, 'autonomous complexes', 'splinter psyches' or 'little people' (Jung 1953, Volume 8). Jung's later work brought him to realise that the 'character' of these different personalities, far from being constituted of idiosyncratic components arising solely from the patient's experience, in fact demonstrated elemental similarities which arose from a collective depth.

It was in people suffering from psychoses that Jung witnessed these components erupting and interfering with conscious mental functioning and which Jung alleged occurred as a result of too wide an abyss between the unconscious treasure-house of images and the conscious process of assimilating and understanding the impulses which motivate our behaviour. The more the mental chasm widens, the more likely that the images from the depths will burst forth upon us in a way thoroughly arresting of all reasonable faculties. This is why Jung was adamant to encourage any process which nurtured and facilitated the methodological admission of unconscious contents into consciousness; for this enabled the sequestered and insensible images of the deeps to be unearthed, observed, wrought, formulated and incorporated into conscious life, rendering neutral their tendency to burst forth pathologically. It would be a misunderstanding, however, to assume Jung believed that therapy should nurture the multiplicity and disorientation of psychological elements, producing people who could not maintain any consistent sense of identity but were this one minute and that the next. Far from this, Jung believed that despite the innate tendency for personal and archetypal characteristics to cluster into complex structures which appeared as distinct personalities, there was an equally strong, or perhaps stronger tendency for the psyche as a whole to hold all these elements in orbit around a single centre, the unifying presence of which is ideally experienced by the patient as overriding the identities of any of the smaller parts.

Jung called the sense of being 'one' in the face of continual disruptions and interruptions from the unconscious the 'Self' and despite diverse beliefs as to the subtle nature of the Self, this term is widely used by psychologists, psychiatrists and psychotherapists from different theoretical and practical fields to denote this 'sense of I' which remains regardless of the transient quality of internal or external circumstances.

But Jung's notion of the Self was more than 'a sense of I'. First, he proposed that as the ego is for the conscious, so the Self is for the unconscious. While the ego acts as the central point around which the feelings and actions of which we are conscious orbit, the Self provides the same centre for all those influences of which we are unaware. He described the Self as the 'most important and most central of archetypes' with 'the significance of a ruler of the inner world' or of 'the collective unconscious' (Jung 1953, Volume 5). Whilst the ego keeps our conscious world of abstract thought and sensible impressions coherent, the Self, we hope, will organise the populace of our deepest mental canyons, it will stop us falling apart at the seams.

To complicate matters, Jung proposed that whilst the Self acts as a centre, it also represents the psyche as a whole, being both the centre and the circumference of the psychic circle and containing the conscious, and therefore along with it the ego; and as we cannot perceive anything but through the ego's faculties, it is in fact impossible to have a complete sense of Self, because the parts cannot comprehend the whole. However, this sense of whole which accommodates but does not yield to the dominance of the parts was, for Jung, something that must nonetheless be forever strived for and is comparable to the Buddhist's search for Enlightenment or the Christian's search for God. Indeed, the search for the Self was, for Jung, as much a spiritual journey as it was a therapeutic procedure. This journey represents our striving for wholeness and unity, the universal search for the true sense of who we are and the promise of a feeling of having found ourselves; indeed Jung at one point defined the Self as the 'God within us'. The Self is a longed-for perspective, a place from which we will be able to see with an inner eye and perceive the order of things. Jung, in naming this centre the

Self, admitted that it 'is no more than a psychological concept, a construct that serves to express an unknowable essence which we cannot grasp as such, since by definition it transcends our powers of comprehension' (Jung 1953, Volume 7).

Jung thus arrived at a conflict between the notion of multiplicity and that of a single cohering Self. By 1959, when Jung was nearing the end of his life, he said that 'so far' he had 'found no stable or definite centre in the unconscious' and had come to believe that no such centre exists. For Jung, the Self had become 'an ideal centre' representing humanity's 'dream of totality' (Jung 1968).

My Self and My Many Selves

In recent years this dream of totality, which remained central to Jung's psychotherapeutic practice, has been publicly questioned, challenged and dismantled by a number of renowned therapists working within the framework of analytical psychology, namely Joseph Redfearn, Michael Fordham and James Hillman. It would be wrong to imply that these therapists share an identical vision or even a common terminology, but underlying the linguistic complexities in which all of their work is couched there is a single fundamental re-visioning of the notion of mental health. In this vision the dream of totality is substituted for a dream of multiplicity. In other words, the tendency for the constituting material of the psyche to fragment into partially autonomous units appearing as discrete personalities with distinct voices which impregnate the 'sense of I' is not viewed as pathological but as the natural and intended state of mental functioning. In this view, the psyche is composed of many 'Is', many voices or many selves which Fordham calls de-integrates, which Redfearn refers to as sub-personalities and which Hillman refrains from naming in any consistent fashion. Common to all is the steering of the therapeutic process towards tolerance of multiplicity. Fordham, for example, says that 'any concept of mental health' must include acknowledgement of the fact that the psyche is 'a periodically unstable system' the growth of which 'must involve periodic experiences of disorder felt as dangerous or even chaotic' (Fordham 1985). Redfearn, meanwhile, has continued the mission of establishing a polycentric vision of the psyche in which it is accepted as a factor of mental health that 'the basic feeling of unity and continuity and of being a person is subject to marked fluctuations and disruptions' by which a person experiences himself or herself not as one person, but as a different person at different times (Redfearn 1985). Further to this, James Hillman's work not only redirects the psychotherapeutic procedure to tolerate multiplicity, he transforms such a goal into the code for a way of life, implying the futility of a search for any kind of exclusive centre. For Hillman no individual can 'provide a norm even for himself' because the psyche is deliberately structured by the grace of the gods 'to save the diversity and autonomy of the psyche from domination by any single power'. Hillman, like Fordham and Redfearn stresses that the manifestation of multiplicity is not a sign of pathology, but asserts that 'because we have come to realise that each of us is normally a flux of figures, we no longer need to be menaced by the notion of multiple personality', such that 'I may see visions and hear voices' and 'I may talk with them and they with each other without at all being insane' (Hillman 1977). Hillman's reference to multiple personality, which is in many contexts perceived as a severe disorder, is a salient provocation which points to the actual clinical context of psychotherapy and is an issue over which the advocates of polycentricity, Hillman particularly, have been questioned and challenged.

Multiple Personality Disorder

Beyond the field of psychotherapy in the wards of psychiatric hospitals, and in the consulting rooms of psychiatrists and clinical psychologists, the notion of being composed of many selves still retains its pathological colouring and has implications of such a nature that any philosophy proposing to nurture such a model of health appears dangerous and morally irresponsible. Many psychiatrists have studied people who have had a tendency to behave as different personalities to such a marked degree of differentiation that one does not remember what the other has done; and some of these cases have involved criminal activity. In the USA, Multiple Personality Syndrome has been the source of considerably extensive investigation by lawyers and psychologists and some have suggested that, because of the lenient consideration with which the United States legal profession treats those diagnosed as mentally ill, intelligent criminals are potentially able to use the deliberate manifestation of multiplicity as a shield from execution or imprisonment.

Hillman refrains from approaching the subjects of criminology, or extreme manifestations of multiplicity which cause pain and suffering to the host. Redfearn on the other hand has recognised that 'many destructive actions' seem to be performed as though 'the person is possessed by a violent subpersonality' or in a state of which he says afterwards 'I don't know what came over me'. But even though Fordham and Redfearn have included clinical material from their own cases to support the process of tolerance towards multiplicity, there is still an epistemological fissure between the research of the various branches of post-Jungian psychology into a polycentric model of health, and the implications of multiple personality in the field of psychiatry and the treatment of psychoses. It should be pointed out, though, that those patients who select or who are referred for psychotherapy as their primary treatment tend not to be those whose 'little people' manifest themselves in behavioural tendencies with criminal or heavily anti-social consequences or who do not remember what one of their selves has done. In fact, one of the most common conditions which emerges in the course of psychotherapy is precisely the reverse; what we might call a monophrenia, a state in which a person becomes stifled by the dominating influence of a single aspect of his or her Self. Redfearn himself says that 'if all one's sub-personalities were spread out like a map or landscape' there would be places 'which were often visited by the conscious "I", and others which would never have been visited'; and many 'people are stuck in one role much of the time, especially if that role has paid dividends in the past' (Redfearn 1985).

It is here that Voice Movement Therapy can offer a primary contribution to psychotherapy, for by facilitating a malleability of vocal timbre which can express a diversity of characteristics, we can facilitate expressively the journey through the selves of which Redfearn speaks. Yet, because vocalisation is a conscious act of composition, the multiplicity of voices can co-exist alongside a stable sense of Self.

Alfred Wolfsohn and the Sounds of Psyche

The idea that the human voice might render psychic contents audible, thereby expanding both the range of voice and the sense of Self was first discovered and investigated by Alfred Wolfsohn.

Alfred Wolfsohn was born in Berlin of Jewish descent in 1896. At the outbreak of World War I he was called to serve as a medic in the front-line trenches during which time he became both horrified and fascinated by the incredible sounds which the adverse conditions and suffering prompted from the voices of dying and wounded soldiers. Like thousands of others, Wolfsohn returned from the war in a state of mental disturbance and was classified as suffering from 'war neurosis' or 'shell-shock'. During the year following the war his illness worsened and he became plagued by aural hallucinations of the extreme vocal sounds which he had heard in the trenches. His inner world became bombarded with a minefield of sounds which remembered the cacophony of the front-line and at the centre of this hallucinated landscape of sound were the pleading screams and groans of the dying.

Wolfsohn became convinced that his illness arose from an intense feeling of guilt at having declined to help a dying comrade for fear of losing his own life, and the voices continued to sound in his mind despite prolonged psychiatric treatment; he felt therefore, that there was no choice but to search for his cure in himself.

Through constant and painful contemplation of his own mental state, Wolfsohn became convinced that if he could actually sing the sounds that haunted his mind he would be able to bring about a cathartic release of the emotion of terror and guilt associated with the voices and by so doing silence them.

In extending the range of his voice and holding in mind the extreme emotive sounds he had heard in the trenches he realised that his voice could express an extensive collage of emotions, moods and characters which embraced not only the dark and agonising sounds of suffering but those of the utmost joy and pleasure. As a result of vocal catharsis, not only did he cure his illness, but he became convinced that there exists a universal human voice of much broader circumference than had hitherto been imagined.

In 1933 a renowned Jewish opera singer and teacher, Paula Salomon-Lindberg, gave Wolfsohn a job teaching singing to some of her younger students which enabled Wolfsohn to embark on the process of passing on to others the results of his own investigations. One of the students who attended his classes in these early years had been a patient of Jungian psychotherapy prior to working vocally with Wolfsohn. She recorded that the road taken towards the development of her voice which she underwent when working with Wolfsohn where the singer arrives at the new, unfamiliar and unknown sound of her voice, to which she listens as though to the voice of a stranger (Newham 1997c), was similar to that taken in following the psychology of Jung.

In 1939, Wolfsohn escaped Germany and fled to London; and when the war was over he gathered a fresh set of students and began teaching his work from a small studio in Golders Green where he achieved the practical realisation of his vision. Through consistent and in-depth work, Wolfsohn enabled his pupils to exceed what they had hitherto believed to be the fixed boundaries of vocal expression. Wolfsohn's intention was not to nurture the diligence and technical proficiency of the 'voice beautiful', but to utilise the potential range of the human voice as a probe and a mirror, investigating and reflecting the many aspects of the human psyche. Therefore, those who took lessons with him committed themselves not only to a thorough psycho-archeology of their psyche, but to the process of acquiring the courage and the ability to express the many aspects of themselves through the voice.

Wolfsohn was particularly inspired by Jung's views on the collective nature of psychic experience which enabled him to consider that the sounds that he had heard and the pain he had endured were not his own, but those of humankind. However, whilst Jung was preoccupied with the pictorial expression of archetypal motifs in dreams, Wolfsohn felt he had discovered a way of making them audible through the sounds of the human voice. An important part of Wolfsohn's work to this end involved a translation of visual dream-images into sound.

Wolfsohn had become particularly interested in an archetype which Jung called the 'shadow' and which represents the dark side of our personality, that which we would never wish to become and which personifies everything that the subject refuses to acknowledge about himself.

For Jung, one of the definitive and universal aspects of the shadow is its animalistic quality, being the sum total of those aspects of our psyche which preserve the residue of an early time in the evolutionary process, a time when the distinction between humanity and animality was not so great. By shadow Jung meant the inferior personality, the lowest levels of which are indistinguishable from the instinctuality of an animal (Jung 1953, Volume 9, Part 2).

The psychological concept of the shadow corresponds to the aesthetic concept of ugliness; and Wolfsohn recognised that if the voice was to be employed as an expression of the true nature of the psyche in its entirety, it would have to establish a connection with the shadow. This meant that the voice had to be permitted to yell, scream, sob, and give voice to the animalistic, primal, preverbal utterances which are part of the rightful expression of the shadow. Wolfsohn's psychologised approach to singing training thus led to the spontaneous emergence of an extraordinary variety of animal sounds which had a very special meaning for each pupil as though a deeper strata of a past evolutionary process had been touched upon and was being relived (Newham 1997c). For his pupils, this was a far cry from singing beautifully. But from this process developed a different kind of beauty which was an authentic expression of the Self.

Wolfsohn was keen to systematically oppose the tradition of specialisation upon which classical singing had been founded and which allotted certain qualities according to gender – soprano, mezzo-soprano and alto for women, and tenor, baritone and bass for men – considering it an unnecessary way of artificially restraining the voice. Wolfsohn thus challenged the popular preconceptions regarding the expressive limits implied and imposed by human gender and drew further support from Jung and the latter's belief in the existence of the archetypes anima and animus. Jung proposed that a man 'has in him a feminine side, an unconscious feminine figure' of which 'he is generally quite unaware' which he called the 'anima', and its counterpart which is the male figure in a woman he called the 'animus' (Jung 1953, Volume 9, Part 1). Wolfsohn further conceived of the idea that the anima and animus in their contra-sexual aspects were potentially audible through the human voice and believed that by giving a voice to the anima or animus they could be projected into sound, confronted audibly and aurally and, finally, accepted and integrated into consciousness. Thus he nurtured a bass voice in women and a soprano voice in men.

Many people became suspicious, not only that Wolfsohn's approach was 'unnatural', but that he was causing damage to his pupils' vocal apparatus. In order to assuage these fears some of the pupils had their voices subjected to scientific measurement whilst producing their extended range. Amongst these students was a young woman called Jenny Johnson who in 1955 had her voice examined by Professor Luchsinger of the Zurich Otolaryngo-logical Clinic using X-ray, high-speed film and a stroboscope. This examination confirmed a range of six octaves and discovered no abnormality in the anatomical structure or physiological functioning of the larynx (Newham 1997c). Luchsinger's discoveries corroborated Wolfsohn's deepest belief that the range of the voice depended not on any exceptional physical virtuosity or on an unnatural or maladjusted anatomy, but on psychological investigation of the deepest regions of the psyche.

Wolfsohn claimed to have found that 'each individual is variously prey to a whole host of psychic inhibitions and conflicts, anxieties and complexes, the elimination of which leads to the opening out of the personality and the voice'. By helping his students to 'overcome their inner tensions and difficulties', Wolfsohn was able to 'loosen the inhibitions' which held their 'personalities as well as their voices in chains' (Newham 1997c).

Wolfsohn wrote to Jung early in 1955 enclosing manuscripts which described his work, but on 3 May 1955 Aniela Jaffe wrote back to say that Jung himself would not be able to take note of his investigations (Newham 1997c). This was a great blow to Wolfsohn who felt that he may never get his work formally appreciated in more established circles. However, the psychotherapeutic benefits of singing and sound-making under Wolfsohn's direction are preserved in the testimony of many of his students who are still living, some of whom are themselves still teaching the work which he pioneered.

When Wolfsohn died, the direction of his work and the leadership of the group which had grown up under him was taken over by an actor called Roy Hart, who had worked with Wolfsohn for over 15 years. What had begun as a therapeutic investigation with performance dimensions now became a theatrical investigation with therapeutic implications as Roy Hart began to steer the work towards presentations of experimental vocal performances. It was from this transition that the Roy Hart Theatre was born.

The Roy Hart Theatre

One of the most radical and significant contributions to vocal work on the interface between therapy and theatre is that contributed by the members of the Roy Hart Theatre, a company which was founded upon the initial research of Alfred Wolfsohn.

Wolfsohn's students had discovered that freeing the voice also liberates other artistic aptitudes and that vocal malleability is a great asset when it comes to producing dramatic presentations. During the later period of his teaching, Wolfsohn had opened the studio doors to the entire clientele of students at any time during the work so that they were able to learn from both the experience of their own process and also from the observation of others and which led to the organic emergence of a working group. Amongst the group was a South African called Roy Hart who had come to England to study as an actor at the Royal Academy of Dramatic Art. Inspired by the performance quality of vocal demonstrations which the pupils did for observers, Roy Hart was keen to develop the work beyond presentations to invited guests for the purposes of demonstrating technique, towards theatre performances which utilised the extended vocal range in a dramatic context which stood in its own right as art; thus he began performing poems and songs using an extended vocal range.

With the death of Wolfsohn in 1962, Roy Hart announced clearly that it was his intention to further the work towards theatre and invited the group to join him in the pursuit of experiments in a new form of vocal dramatics. The 'Alfred Wolfsohn Voice Research Centre' now became the 'Roy Hart Theatre' and what had begun with small voice demonstrations slowly took the shape of theatrical performances. All members of the Roy Hart Theatre – particularly Roy Hart himself – became renowned for their incredible ability to refract their voices through every contour of the sound prism, producing an incredible acoustic spectrum from the bleak to the divine. In 1969, the composer Peter Maxwell-Davies composed a full length piece for Roy Hart called *Eight Songs for a Mad King* with subsequent performances given internationally and in response to which Hart was described as an artist who commands all the voices of the human register – ranging from the deepest bass to the highest soprano.

Many reviewers described the performances of the Roy Hart Theatre as a psychological experience and there was recognition of the psychological implications of the work not only from the theatre profession, but from psychotherapeutic circles also. During the 1960s and early 1970s Hart and the company presented their research in the form of lectures and demonstrations at psychotherapy and arts therapy conferences all over the world.

When Roy Hart took over the work initiated by Alfred Wolfsohn, he was drawing on a long tradition of twentieth-century avant-garde theatre which had become increasingly fascinated with the subject of the human voice. Indeed, vocal expression is as central to the development of theatre in the twentieth century as it is to the development of archetypal psychology. It is therefore towards this subject that I will now turn my attention.

CHAPTER 2

The Psyche on Stage
Voice and Therapy in European Theatre

Voice and Therapy in the Rehearsal Studio

Whilst the notion of a dramatic cast of characters with specific voices has been central to the development of a Jungian paradigm of the psyche, so the use of voice to give dramatic expression to the polyphonic and multifaceted nature of the psyche has been central to the development of twentieth-century theatre. The history of Western theatre contains astoundingly rich and consistent investigations into the way vocal expression can communicate the nature of the psyche to an audience. Furthermore, the experimental theatre has contributed more to the practical exploration of the vocal instrument than any other subject.

The Elocutionists

During the eighteenth century the hitherto prevailing neoclassic style of acting and vocal delivery, consisting of pantomimical and melodramatic gesture, was challenged and reformed by the actor David Garrick. Through his acting style, he introduced a simpler, more measured vocal delivery that focused on a precision of diction which sought to more properly represent the turns of thought underlying the text in the theatre. It was to this theatre that the elocution teachers Thomas Sheridan and John Walker turned in their search for models of vocal delivery which could inform their pedagogical principles. The art of elocution was founded on a precision of distinct articulation and pronunciation with punctilious observation of emphasis and of rests or pauses of the voice, accompanied by expressive looks and descriptive gestures.

Then, in 1827, the American James Rush attempted to provide a scientific description of vocal physiology and a system for notating speech sounds, whilst simultaneously merging philosophy, biology and art in an attempt to explain the human condition. The American writer, actor and teacher James Murdoch, who was tutored by Rush, sought to carry on his work through his own teaching, and in so doing became a leader of the American elocutionary movement for over 50 years. Moreover, a number of Murdoch's pupils went on to become influential teachers of the elocution movement in the US educational establishments of the nineteenth century which formed the basis for the vocal delivery of America's great actors of the period such as Charlotte Cushman, Mary Ann Duff and Edwin Booth, whose voices of orotund tones and pear-shaped vowels, consciously sculptured cadence and poetic rhythm suited the classic theatre popular at the time. Towards the end of the nineteenth century, however, things began to change, partly due to the American Silas Curry.

Curry rejected much of the mechanistic and didactic techniques which had descended from Rush's approach and became fascinated with the connection between mind, body and voice. In fact, Curry became the first teacher in America to proclaim that the inner motivations of the mind must be studied and trained in tandem with its outward expression through movement and sound. This new approach to voice and speech lent itself to the emerging realism in the theatre. However, this focus on the inner truth behind the words was, in many ways, countermanded by a fresh force or emphasis on the outer mechanics of expression, under the title of a new science: phonetics.

Phonetics

Phonetics is the study of speech sounds as formed by the mechanical movements of physiological components such as tongue, lips and teeth. It was the British Henry Sweet who in the late nineteenth century first proclaimed the educational virtues of phonetics, pointing out its use in learning foreign languages and in creating a uniformity of pronunciation within a given language. The most renowned American proponent of this phonetic approach to standardising speech was Margaret Prendergast McClean, who influenced speech training in schools, universities and drama colleges. Her aim was to use phonetic science to remove the regional variation from speech and produce a standard American dialect called Transatlantic. This borrowed from standard British pronunciations and sought to provide a form of enunciation which did not reveal the ethnic, regional, geographical or cultural origins of the speaker. The influence of this training can be heard in the speech of a number of film actors including Bette

Davis, Katherine Hepburn and Tyrone Power. Both the Standard English, or Received Pronunciation, and the Transatlantic mode of speaking became associated, however, not with a neutral predicament but with the upper classes, the educated and the rich.

The phonetic approach to voice training encouraged a perception of speech as a sociological phenomenon, that is to say the precision, diction and elocution of the spoken word was taken to be directly proportional to a person's intelligence, status and social worth. Probably the most well-known example of an equation between speech and social standing is revealed in the story of Eliza Doolittle as told in Shaw's *Pygmalion* and whose transformation from a 'sloppy speaker' to a 'posh speaker' is seen to be equivalent and directly related to her transformation from a member of a lower social class to a higher one. Such an understanding of the sociological function of speech is innately bound to a certain puritanical view of the English language where certain acoustic articulations are generated, inculcated and preserved by the privileged members of society who tend to be moneyed, physically able and educated. The perpetuation of this so-called superior etiquette in the manner of speaking has been the responsibility of elocution teachers in both England and America.

Melodrama

Despite the various schools of articulate inner truth, most popular nine-teenth-century European theatre was prosaic in language, histrionic in gesture, decorative in scenic style and declamatory in utterance. This was a theatre which presented a world of exaggerated emotion, heightened atmospheres and a poetic inflation of mood, narrative and character. Such a theatre required a vocal style of delivery that could make audient the grandiose experience, the intense mood and the romantic sentiment of the world which it portrayed. The great voices which dominated the stage of the nineteenth century served a particular kind of literary drama, such as the romantic plays of Alexander Dumas and Victor Hugo, the elaborate poetry and rhythmic verse of Shakespeare and above all, the genre of theatre known as melodrama which was proliferate during this period.

Commonly, the word melodrama denotes a style of dramatic performance, extremely popular in the nineteenth century, where choreographically stylised movement, graphic depiction of emotion and declamatory vocal enunciation portrayed sensational scenarios in which the good are ensnared by the clutches of evil as the audience await the inevitable and guaranteeable triumph of justice. The style of vocal delivery which served this theatre was somewhere between singing and speaking. It was a declaiming in which prosody and intonation drifted towards melodic composition and verbal intensities came close to musical crescendos.

The term *melodrama*, which to theatre practitioners refers to this style of drama, also denotes a musical genre in which a vocalist speaks or declaims a poem, text or libretto to the accompaniment of music, sometimes in silent pauses between melodic phrases and at others simultaneous with the music. Many great composers also wrote melodramas, including Mozart, and Beethoven; and there have also been classical operas with melodramatic sections in which the vocalist speaks to musical accompaniment rather than sings.

In melodrama, the words were not set to a musical score and the vocalist was therefore completely free from the demands of pitch, register, voice quality and note value, and able to work as a declaimer, an orator, an actor, but was not required to display the skills of a singer or musician. Consequently, many composers simply laid text over a musical score and left it to the performer's discretion as to how to declaim it. The manner of declaiming used by the vocalist in musical melodrama is comparable to the form of vocal articulation used by actors on the theatrical stage during the nineteenth century which housed romantic and exaggerated scenarios, acoustic sound effects simulating thunder and lightning which emerged from behind the elaborately coloured scenery, and an acting style that was entirely in keeping with such sensationalism.

There were a number of particularly renowned disseminators of this style such as the American Edwin Forrest whose voice was described as 'tremendous in its sustained crescendo swell and crashing force of utterance' which 'surged and roared like the angry sea' as it 'reached its boiling, seething climax, in which the serpent hiss of hate was heard', 'it was like the falls of Niagara, in its tremendous down-sweeping cadence; it was a whirlwind, a tornado, a cataract of illimitable rage' (Newham 1997b, p.357).

The Naturalistic Utterance

Towards the end of the nineteenth century an avalanche of artistic sensibilities caused a pan-European and transatlantic shift in theatre away from declamatory romantic sensationalism, towards an attempted more truthful replication of actual life behaviours, which was instigated and compounded by a twofold development within both the novel and dramatic literature. First, the content of literature moved away from romantic and melodramatic scenarios towards the realism of sociopolitical reality. It was the French novelist Émile Zola who in the 1870s first proclaimed the need for truthful representation in the literary arts; and the harsh realities of European social life, particularly the plight of the downtrodden Russian peasant, were also portrayed by Leo Tolstoy. In Germany, meanwhile, Gerhart Hauptmann portrayed the exhausting attempt of the poor and disenfranchised to escape from the bleakness of their social surroundings. The second development in literature, was the development of a realistic dramatic text in which the style of dialogue moved towards the naturalism of everyday discourse without the hitherto dominance of poetic embellishment of verse, rhyme and metre. One of the effects of this development was to completely change the way the actor used the voice upon the stage.

In Norway, for example, the poet Henrik Ibsen sought to portray an inner condition rather than an outer circumstance, which required a subtlety of vocal delivery which could intimate the gentle pulse of an internal psychic reality. The plays of Ibsen, Turgenev and Chekhov also required a mode of delivery that did justice to writing which was conversational and akin to the way people speak in the garden, on the street and in the drawing room. Many of these plays relied on a kind of impressionistic build up of effects from a multitude of minute details in which stumblings and stammerings, grunts and sighs and sustained silences drew attention to the meaning inherent in what was not overtly said. It required the audience to listen to a 'subtext', an 'undertone', a hidden language of deeper desire that lay beneath that which the characters were able to express verbally in their social context. And this second unspoken dialogue was facilitated by various devices including the cadences of vocal expression.

Because this style of dialogue and human representation usually went hand in hand with a realistic representation of society, with its hypocrisies and blemishes, the plays of the naturalistic school were often censored and reviewed harshly. In response to this, a number of private theatre clubs or societies were founded where new plays of the naturalistic style could be played to receptive audiences. One of the most famous of these was the French Théâtre Libre, where the naturalist experimenter André Antoine produced new plays by unknown writers using amateur actors. Antoine broke with many of the presiding performance traditions which had been the very constitution of the actor's art, encouraged a simple undeclaimed vocal style of delivery and attempted to create for the audience the illusion of eavesdropping in on someone's private affair.

The Actor's Method of Naturalism

One of the famous private societies which produced naturalistic plays, censored in the main frame of conventional theatre, was the Moscow Art Theatre where the Russian theatre director Constantin Stanislavski set himself the task of devising a methodological approach to training actors in how to manifest and embody the naturalistic vision of dramatic literature that elevated the elusive, implied, elliptical and the obtuse.

To reflect the truth of human discourse and of the human condition meant allowing dialogue to retain its incompleteness, its manifold implications and dual meanings, its inherent conflicts of desire, its double-binds and ambivalences. Within Stanislavski's system, careful attention was given to allowing the voice to contain both the text and the subtext. For, Stanislavski felt that it was in the subtle twists and turns of the vocal dimension to speech that the intricacy and ambiguity of meaning was communicable to an attentive audience.

In 1923 the Moscow Art Theatre toured America, exposing audiences and actors to the system of Stanislavski in action; and in 1924 the principles of his method were taught by former members of the theatre at the American laboratory theatre in New York. It was at these classes that Lee Strasberg first experienced the techniques which he adapted to form the Strasberg Method which was to influence a generation of American actors, most notably Marlon Brando.

In the Americanised method approach, actors mumbled, spoke whilst eating and attempted to find the most naturalistic way of behaving which meant letting the voice follow the reality of the inner life. With the elocutionist and phonetic approach no longer suited to the emerging school of realistic plays being written for the theatre, and with audiences seeking naturalism of enunciation even in the classic works of Shakespeare, a new approach to training the voice became necessary.

Strindberg: External Replication to Inner Truth

Whilst Stanislavski experimented in Moscow, the Swedish writer August Strindberg formed his own society in Copenhagen where he tried to use naturalism to expose the richness of the psyche. Strindberg became involved in portraying the nature of the inner psychic world. His characters were conglomerations of past and present stages of civilisation patched together as is – according to Strindberg – the human soul. Strindberg wanted to avoid mathematically-constructed dialogue and allow the characters' minds to work irregularly, as he believed people's minds worked in real life.

This inevitable bridge from naturalism as a replication of life's behaviours to naturalism as a truthful portrayal of the way that life is experienced subjectively and intrapsychically, exemplified in Strindberg's writing, symbolised a widespread move amongst writers to reach a deeper level of reality than the deceptive appearances of replicated discourse and to embody the inner nature of archetypal man in concrete symbols rather than perpetrate the naturalistic depiction of socially defined individuals. Thus the notion of naturalism was broadened to include any form which represents the truth of inner world by tracing every nuance of the psyche. Thus, naturalism carried the seeds of the future within it and led to a number of fresh waves or movements.

Symbolism and Silence

One of the fresh artistic waves which challenged the precepts of naturalism and realism was symbolism; and the playwright who became the embodiment of the new symbolist trend was Maurice Maeterlinck, a Belgian poet whose plays were first staged at the experimental Théâtre d'artin in 1891. Maeterlinck worked towards a theatre of silence proclaiming that puppets make the ideal actors, and he sought to encourage his actors to abandon realistic expression for a musically structured gesture. Here, the emphasis was placed on expressive tone and pitch in speaking rather than on the sense of what was said. One of the actors who had helped realise Maeterlinck's vision was Aurélien Lugné-Poë who, following his success as an actor in Maeterlinck's plays, launched his own company, the Théâtre de l'Oeuvre, which he wanted to be a temple to Symbolist Drama and at which Alfred Jarry's slapstick and absurd theatre production *Ubu roi* was performed in December 1896.

Alfred Jarry was an absinthe drinker, a philosopher, an eccentric and a relentless practical joker. His performance, *Ubu roi,* had begun as a satirical lampoon of an unpopular school teacher and developed into a savage attack on the greed and power-crazed obsessions of the French bourgeois. The opening word of this performance was 'merdre', that is a slightly mispronounced 'shit'. It was probably the first time this taboo word had been heard upon the French stage. The performance provoked uproar in the audience whose riotous cacophony brought the action to a halt and made the dialogue almost inaudible. It played for only two nights, but in two performances Jarry had made history.

Futurism

In addition to hosting the outlandish Alfred Jarry, France was also the home of the wealthy Italian poet, Filippo Tommaso Marinetti who published a manifesto in the Parisian daily newspaper Le Figaro which announced the arrival of Futurism and which described the new art of 'declamation' that was to be the trademark of Futurist performance. Marinetti asserted that the new form of declaiming should completely dehumanise the performer, systematically destroying every naturalistic nuance. The first practical demonstrations of this art were in the performances of free verse plays performed in 1914 in which the performers declaimed the words whilst the author played the piano, banged drums and simulated cannon fire. Concurrently, a number of home-made 'noise instruments' were played including a saw with pieces of tin attached. After witnessing one of the Futurist performances, the musician and experimentalist Luigi Russolo became convinced that mechanised noises were a viable form of music and wrote his manifesto The Arts of Noises. His intention was to combine the noises of trams, trains, shouting crowds and exploding motors; and he created a futurist orchestra of specially constructed boxes which made such sounds at the turn of the handle. According to Russolo, at least thirty thousand diverse noises were possible. Russolo's ideas had a significant effect on the later composer John Cage who had studied composition with Schoenberg in the mid-1930s. Cage was fascinated in the subject of noise and in his early performances his 'musicians' played beer bottles, flowerpots, cowbells and other found objects expanding the musical framework to incorporate that which may in other circumstances be regarded as unmusical noise.

Futurism also took hold in Russia where the deconstruction of language into a non-sense or sense-free language was encapsulated in the work of the poet Vladimir Mayakovsky who provoked audiences with his readings and self-proclaimed genius. During the second two decades of the twentieth century a number of poets in Russia experimented with poetic language in an attempt to disintegrate concept, words and musical harmony and replace them with a variety of vocal sounds which had an emotional impact without having any syntactical sense. All of this futuristic work involved an attack on grammar and syntax and placed the emphasis on sonic and pictorial qualities of words.

Dada

Another radical and disruptive attack on artistic convention occurred in Zurich where a group of artists presented spectacles designed to be anti-art. Their meeting place and platform was the Cabaret Voltaire founded on 5 February 1916 and their movement was named Dada out of which surrealism is said to have grown.

It was here, at the cabaret, that they experimented with a new species of verse without words or 'sound poems' which they composed according to the acoustic properties of vowels and consonants to produce phrases such as 'glandridi glassala tuffm i zimbrabim'. Meanwhile, in 1920s Paris, where Picasso was painting, where Cocteau was experimenting with dream images in film and theatre, the composer Erik Satie, in the final years of his life, was experimenting with the potential musical noise of typewriters, sirens, aeroplane propellers and Morse tappers.

The Experimental Pioneers

The vitality of the growing avant-garde influenced the French poetic visionary Antonin Artaud who spent the first half of the twentieth century oscillating between obsessional and pioneering ponderances on the potential of the theatre to provoke the most archetypal strata of the human condition and debilitating periods of mental illness.

Central to Artaud's quest was the search for a non-verbal use of the voice to communicate fundamental aspects of the human condition. And the range of vocal delivery styles used in theatre groups since the 1960s which used sounds rather than words, screams and cries rather than speech, owed much to the original impetus provided by his writings.

Artaud, who admired the acting of Lugné-Poë, being particularly fascinated by his surprising changes of voice and his inflamed glances, sought to liberate Western theatre from what he described as the 'exclusive dictatorship of words'. Reacting against the great wave of realistic plays that had swept Europe, Artaud criticised the theatre for reducing what he regarded as the mysteriously unapproachable and evasive images of the human psyche to the level of everyday conversation and linguistic discourse.

For Artaud, the written text and the spoken word of the actor had turned theatre into an arena for every day social conflicts. Artaud believed that theatre should approach those subjects for which speech is inadequate or is unable to express, rediscovering the figures which gave expression to archetypal symbols. This theatre was to be not verbal but vocal, utilising a genuine physical language, no longer based on words but on signs formed through the combination of objects, silence, shouts and rhythms which would be a powerful appeal through illustration to those powers which return the mind to the origins of its inner struggles. He thought that the theatre, in seeking to realise this, should return to the idea of poetry underlying the myths told by the great tragedians of ancient times.

It was the focus on voice combined with the use of myth that influenced a chain of theatre practitioners who had studied and admired Artaud, including Peter Brook, for whom the twentieth-century British theatre was restrained from dealing with such archetypal images by an unceasing adherence to the eloquent articulation of text. By the same token, Brook perceived the opera to be deprived of its potential potency by an overly scrutinising attention to the artificial formal structures of music.

The means by which Brook sought to revive the natural expressive function of the human voice was to set up experimental theatre workshops at the Royal Shakespeare Company in the early 1960s in which he required of his actors that they communicate to an audience without the use of words. It was here that Brook exercised his determination to investigate the degree to which Artaud's pleas might be fulfilled. Encouraged by his discoveries, Brook continued with his vocal experiments when he collaborated with the writer Ted Hughes to devise a production of *Oedipus* which used chants based on those uttered by the Maori peoples of New Zealand and irregular breathing rhythms derived from a recording of a medicine man in a trance. Brook became so intrigued by these experiments into the nature of vocal sound that he founded the International Theatre Research Centre in Paris, a company of actors of different nationalities, many of whom were prevented from talking to one another by a language barrier and where the theme of the first year's work was a study of structures of sounds. The motivation was to discover vocal utterances which could communicate the essence of the great myths and archetypes which exposed the fabric of the collective unconscious.

Later, in 1972, Brook set off with his actors to see if it was possible to communicate with people of the tribal communities of Africa through such a non-linguistic vocal code, seeking to create a work of theatre that could be accessible to everyone wherever it was played and discover whether the collective unconscious can be tapped in sound.

During the African journey Brook's troupe encountered the Peuhl tribe, and wondered how it would be possible for the actors and the local tribal members, who did not speak each other's language, to communicate and share a common experience. Brook's first idea was for the acting troop to sing a song, but the Peuhls were not interested, so Brook tried asking his group to make an 'ah' sound. In response, the Peuhls joined the sound and in exchange sang their songs. Brook felt at last that he was on the right road in the search for a universal language.

Whilst Peter Brook was searching for a universal language of sounds at Stratford, in Paris and in Africa, another theatre director called Jerzy Grotowski was researching a similar area in Poland. In 1959 Grotowski became director of a tiny theatre in Opole, Poland called the Theatre of Thirteen Rows. In this theatre in one of the poorest countries in Europe, a group of actors came together to explore the way in which the images of their own collective unconscious could be expressed through the body and the voice, without recourse to the spoken word. They sought, like Artaud, to reach an audience, not through the narrative intrigues of everyday plots, but through an expression of the archetypes which reflect the nature of every man and woman.

In their production of *Akropolis*, which premiered in October 1962, all means of vocal expression was used, starting from the confused babbling of the very small child, including the most sophisticated oratorical recitation as well as inarticulate groans, animal roars, tender folk-songs, liturgical chants, dialects and declamation of poetry which aimed to stimulate the memory of all forms of language. Above all else, Grotowski's group of devout actors became known for their revolutionary work on vocal expression.

The use of non-verbal voice in these productions was part of Grotowski's investigation into the use of the actor's own psychological material as the substance of performance and his work was intricately and overtly bound up with a belief in the ability of a human being to physically and vocally express aspects of the psyche, including those aspects which are buried in the collective unconscious, without recourse to words. Grotowski wanted to build a theatre where nothing was represented or shown, but where the actors participate in a ceremony which releases the collective unconscious. In Grotowski's scheme of things, the actor had to be able to draw from his psyche images of a personal and collective significance and give them form through the motion of the body and the sound of the voice.

Grotowski's ultimate aim was to effect in the actor change and growth, transformation and rebirth in order that the actor, in turn, could entice a similar development in the audience. He sought to bring actor and audience momentarily into contact with the deepest levels within themselves so that they may, as a result of touching those depths, be changed forever. It was for this reason that Grotowski chose old master works based on timeless narratives as subjects for his productions, for he believed that they embodied myths and images powerful and universal enough to function as archetypes, which could penetrate beneath the apparently divisive and individual structure of the Western psyche, and evoke a spontaneous, collective, internal response. Grotowski felt that in order that the spectator may be stimulated into self-analysis when confronted with the actor, there must be some common ground already existing in both of them, something they can either dismiss in one gesture or jointly worship. For him, this common ground was provided by the myths which he believed were not an invention of the mind but inherited. Grotowski's actors drew images out from the depths of the unconscious with the aim of healing. What Grotowski asks of the actor therefore is that he confront the mythical characters within himself and offer the result of that encounter to an audience.

Grotowski, like Artaud, did not consider the text to be primary, but pursued the possibility of creating 'ideograms' made up of sounds and gestures which evoke associations in the psyche of the audience. But, for Grotowski, there was, between the psychic image and the bodily and vocal expression, a series of inhibitions, resistances and blocks which prevent transformation from one to the other and it was these obstacles that his acting exercises set out to remove. Grotowski felt that the education of an actor in his theatre was not a matter of teaching him something but an attempt to eliminate his organism's resistance to this psychic process, the result being freedom from the time-lapse between inner impulse and outer reaction. Training for Grotowski was not a collection of skills but an eradication of blocks which he proposed leads to a liberation from complexes in much the same way as psychotherapy. In rediscovering the power of mythical tales told not only through language but through the expressive power of the human voice, Grotowski reclaimed the therapeutic role of theatre which had been so fundamental to Greek tragedy and upon which Freud built his original cathartic method.

During the early 1960s, Jerzy Grotowski had worked with an assistant called Eugenio Barba who in 1964 founded his own company in Denmark called Odin Theatre, using applicants who had been refused a place at traditional theatre school. The work of Odin now constitutes an internationally influential body of work, known as Theatre Anthropology, the aim of which is to study the cultural and technical foundations upon which different styles, traditions and genres of performance are based. During his time in Poland, Barba helped Grotowski design the sound montage for a production. Barba thus took with him to Denmark an interest in sound, particularly those made by the human voice.

Odin has drawn actors from many countries and the actors do not share a common mother tongue which has led to experiments where, like Brook's group, they have devised pieces based upon the use of their own unique self-created language. All of Barba's productions have a complex vocal score consisting of songs, naturalistic dialogue, languages from different countries, chants, incantations and vocables, in which the voice is used as a musical instrument. Like the theatre of Grotowski, Barba's process is one in which the experience of the actor is revered as central and the dynamic relationships between company members is drawn upon in the rehearsal process.

Artaud and Grotowski also influenced the research of Richard Schechner who founded the New York-based Performance Group in 1967. Schechner wanted to develop a mode of theatre which mirrored participatory rituals indigenous to many non-Western communities; and in this envisioned theatre the established centrality of narrative and character was to be replaced by the ritual image. Schechner further believed that part of the power of such ritual theatre lay in a deep level of communication and expression that was beyond the realm of speech.

Neither Artaud, Brook, Grotowski, Barba nor Schechner were clinically trained or qualified as therapists; yet their work on the human voice was deeply rooted in a respect for the intimate connection between vocal sound and soul. Their field of enquiry was not dramatherapy but vocal theatre which had therapeutic implications. However, the implications of their work were equally relevant to the field of anthropology, performance, literature and mythology. In many ways they returned the notion of therapy to the arts, from which it had been extracted. Such work is therefore significant not only because of its content but because of its form; it reveals how the artistic process can be innately life enhancing without need for a clinical or therapeutic context or explanation in order to qualify it or legitimate its value.

In this day, where there is an ever-increasing momentum towards a clinification of the arts in order to validate their therapeutic application, the work of these practitioners can provide inspiration. And, the fact the voice was central to the investigations of twentieth-century experimental theatre is a significant inspiration for those working in the therapeutic arena who wish to use vocal expression as a dynamic means to personal transformation.

Augusto Boal and the Political Voice

The voice is the means by which we assert our rights in the world, it is a metaphor for our democratic necessity and a medium of expression for our rightful demands. A contemporary theatre practitioner whose work belongs in the tradition of twentieth-century avant-garde, which was originally modelled on a sociopolitical approach to the voice, and to whom the political concept of voice is still a central working component is the Brazilian theatre director and workshop leader Augusto Boal.

Boal began developing a body of work known as The Theatre of the Oppressed in the 1950s when the aim of his work was to mobilise audiences and participants towards an activist stance against Brazil's widespread corruption and oppression of the poor. Central to the work was 'Forum Theatre' where scenes would be presented to an audience who would be permitted to intervene either by directing the actors or by acting themselves, thereby empowering one another to shape and direct the action. Brazil had a military coup in 1964 and again in 1968 and Boal used this theatre work to challenge the harsh conditions of dictatorship. He was then gaoled in 1971 where he was tortured and on his release he moved to Argentina where he resided until 1976. It was here that Boal developed 'Image Theatre' where the human body is used as an expressive tool to represent, non-verbally, a wide repertoire of feelings, ideas, and attitudes. Forbidden to take part in activist theatre by the Argentinean regime, Boal developed 'Invisible Theatre'. These were scenes played out by actors in public spaces in such a way that the audience did not realise they were watching a performance. However, finding it impossible to work, Boal withdrew from theatre activity and sought exile in Europe.

In South America, Boal's work was designed to mobilise people to stand up to what he termed the 'cop in the streets', that is the actual external social violence and pressure of social reality. However, in Europe, workshop participants brought internal problems of psychic fragmentation, selflessness and a host of psychological struggles. At first Boal was frustrated by these oppressions which seemed insignificant when compared to the social hardships he had been confronted with in South America. However, influenced somewhat by his wife who later became a psychoanalyst in France, Boal began to conceive of the 'cop in the head'; that is the introjected and internal voices of oppression absorbed from society, parents, teachers and suspect moral values which continued to plague the adult. Boal's sociopolitical theatre techniques thus took on a psychotherapeutic dimension and his workshops were presented, in many cases, as therapeutic processes. Boal describes his work as a 'psycho-theatre', a realm where theatre and therapy overlap; and in this theatre catharsis for Boal means a purging of those detrimental blocks which inhibit positive social and political action.

Robert Wilson and the Deaf Boy's Scream

Another practitioner who has investigated the inner psychic world of individuals and at the same time acted politically in giving marginalised individuals a central place upon the stage is Robert Wilson.

Robert Wilson was born in Texas in 1941 and as a child suffered from a severe speech impediment which made spoken language difficult to master. In addition to his own handicap, he witnessed the suffering of his sister who was born with a skeletal deformity of the legs and who, for the first 5 years of her life, had to have a series of operations during which her bones were broken and reset to enable her to walk. Wilson's proximity to disability was to have a profound effect on the development of his work as an adult.

At the age of 17, Wilson met an elderly dance instructor, Bird Hoffman, who worked with him over a period of three months encouraging him to relax and release the tensions in his body through movement exercises after which his speech impediment disappeared. The lessons he had learned from Bird Hoffman, which had enabled his own physical liberation, were later applied to his performance work where he was seeking to make public his own process of physical and energetic exploration. In 1966 Wilson began facilitating therapeutic workshops focusing on psychosomatic issues which he conducted with adults and with young, often handicapped, children and which culminated in performances which were presented in construction sites, in churches, in garages or in vacant lots.

Influenced by his exposure to the dance work of Merce Cunningham and Martha Graham, the performance styles of the Judson Dance theatre, particularly the work of Kenneth King and Meredith Monk, as well as the theatrical 'Happenings' staged around New York, the artistic environment of New York in the early 1960s shaped the aesthetics of his theatre as he began to create performances with adult friends and followers who were beginning to gather around him. The lessons learned from the special needs of those in the workshops combined with the influence of other contemporaries thus enabled Wilson to develop a non-narrative image-orientated theatre. In actuality, the workshops in psychosomatic therapy designed to offer a healing process through participation in artistic process did not differ greatly from his theatre workshops which were designed to offer an audience an insight into the psychic reality of each performer, showing not a make-believe character represented by an actor but revealing the performers as themselves. In his therapeutic workshops, Wilson provided movement exercises for participants and at the same time learned from their particular ways of expression, communication and sensibility which he then applied to his theatre workshops and performances which from the early stages had been influenced to a great extent by his work with exceptional children.

Central to Wilson's investigations was his work with Raymond Andrews, a young boy who was almost totally deaf, had no command of language but who vocalised sounds, and with whom Wilson achieved a radical integration of therapy into theatre. Wilson felt that Andrews possessed a special sensibility and unusual ways of communicating which provided a rich alternative and inspiration for the work. For Andrews demonstrated an ability to be exceedingly and exceptionally sensitive to the feelings of others, but he perceived and transmitted messages through kinetic, or kinesthetic awareness rather than through discursive, or verbal dialogue. In children such as Andrews, Wilson sensed not only a deep, special talent but channels usually unknown for establishing lines of communication.

Wilson brought other performers into Andrews' world in which Wilson and the performers attempted to learn his language of sounds and gestures by imitating him. Then, having acquired Andrews' language of non-verbal communication, the troupe constructed a theatre performance which had hardly any words but which dealt almost entirely in images and in sounds like the ones Andrews made. In later performances, Wilson's use of his own voice aimed to show the way that the thoughts of the mind often flow in several directions at once aiming to communicate the idea that verbal discourse cannot adequately provide or express insight. Wilson thus worked his voice through an array of sounds which gave an impression of the dream-like world of the psyche.

From Experiment to Method, From Theatre to Therapy

The work of those like Robert Wilson, Peter Brook, Jerzy Grotowski and Eugenio Barba provided the avant-garde backdrop against which the Roy Hart Theatre turned the work of Alfred Wolfsohn – whom I introduced in the previous chapter – from a therapeutic mission into a theatrical one. Indeed the combined work of Wolfsohn and Hart perhaps represents the most consistent, radical and significant contribution to vocal work on the interface between therapy and theatre. And this work may be seen in the context of a vast spectrum of vocal investigation which underpinned the experimental theatre throughout the twentieth century.

This research and investigation, which I have outlined in this chapter, would seem to verify that the human voice has been recognised as a major channel for authentic human expression. In addition, the realm of theatre has found itself very close to the realm of therapy in its desire to find a means to communicate the authentic essence of the human condition to an audience. And the voice has been a primary tool in this search.

However, in order to take the next step towards incorporating the dramatic use of voice into the arena of a contemporary artistically orientated therapy, it is necessary to go some way towards systematising the use of the vocal instrument in order that its therapeutic applications can be disseminated. One of the problems with the result of the avant-garde investigation of voice is that little has been left in the way of recorded models, techniques and integrated methodologies which can be passed on to those who have not experienced participation in avant-garde theatre practices.

It has been my focus to contribute to the incorporation of dramatic vocal expression into therapy by formulating a system which enables the human voice to be understood, utilised and applied within an Expressive Arts Therapy paradigm. It is a system which is at once grounded in both physiology and creativity and I shall present this system in the following chapter.

CHAPTER 3

The Ingredients of Voice
The Voice Movement Therapy System and the Dramatic Voice

The Ingredients of Voice

Every human voice is produced in the same way, yet every human voice is unique. The sound of a person's voice is like an acoustic fingerprint which carries their identity; and often our reactions to someone's voice are extremely subjective. Some voices attract us and others repel; some voices stimulate our agitation whilst others calm and soothe; some voices dominate with authority and others sound servile and sycophantic; some voices befriend and others contend; some voices we like and others we do not. Yet, rarely do we take the time to consider exactly what it is in a certain voice that provokes our reactions. Without this understanding, we cannot really transcend our subjective judgements and gain insight into the psychology of vocal sound; and the best way to understand the voice is to break it down into the separate acoustic ingredients which combine to create vocal sound and learn how these ingredients are produced.

The human voice is made up of a set of ingredients which combine in different degrees to produce an infinite range of sounds; and there are ten basic ingredients which all voices possess. Our subjective reactions to voices are usually based on a response to these ingredients, just as our reactions to food are based on a response to the taste of specific ingredients which flavour the meal. By understanding the habitual recipe which makes up our own voice, we can make changes and choices, increasing the amount of one ingredient and decreasing the presence of another as we wish. Understanding the ingredients of the voice is therefore useful as a tool with which to analyse other voices and as a guide in the evolution of our own voice towards increasing malleability.

Each vocal ingredient also carries within it certain psychological implications. Just as we might choose to add or subtract specific herbs and spices to a recipe in order to create particular healing results, so the addition and subtraction of specific vocal ingredients can help to heal particular issues. However, in order to achieve this, we have to learn to access the ingredients, and this is made easier by the knowledge of how they are produced.

The ten ingredients of the voice according to the Voice Movement Therapy system are:

- Loudness
- Pitch
- Pitch fluctuation
- Register
- Harmonic timbre
- Nasality
- Free air
- Attack
- Disruption
- Articulation.

The following is a concise description of the nature of each ingredient and its main psychological pertinence. I have presented this system in *Using Voice and Song in Therapy* (Newham 1999b) with reference to the singing voice. I have also described its physiological foundations in more detail in *Therapeutic Voicework* (Newham 1997b). The ingredients of the voice remain stable and constant throughout different aspects of Voice Movement Therapy and they are interconnected through the physiological mechanisms by which they are produced. However, the ingredients do not relate to one another in any particular order and can be introduced to clients in any sequence.

Ingredient One: Loudness

Running from the lips to the lungs is a long elastic tube. This tube begins at the lips, opens out to become the mouth, curls downwards at the throat to become the pharynx which runs into the next section, known as the larynx, before turning into the trachea which, in the centre of the chest, splits into two tubes, one running into each lung. When we breathe in, air passes down this tube, inflating the lungs. When we breathe out, air passes up through this tube in the opposite direction, deflating the lungs. We shall call the part of this tube which extends from the lips to the larynx the voice tube (Figure 3.1).

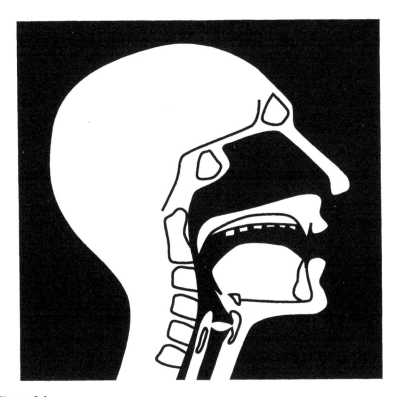

Figure 3.1

Laying stretched out in the larynx are two flaps of tissue called the vocal cords. During normal breathing, the vocal cords lie at rest, one each side of the larynx, like an open pair of curtains allowing air to pass freely through a window. The window between the two vocal cords through which the air passes is called the glottis (Figure 3.2a). There are times, however, when we draw these vocal cords tightly shut, preventing air from passing through the tube in either direction. We often do this momentarily when lifting or moving a heavy object (Figure 3.2b).

(a)

(b)

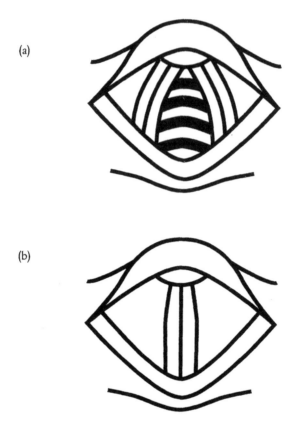

Figure 3.2

The sound of the human voice is produced by the very rapid opening and closing of the vocal cords hundreds of times per second; this is often referred to as the vibration of the vocal cords. During this vibration the two vocal cords hit each other regularly like two hands clapping at great speed. When the vocal cords vibrate in this way they produce a note, just as a string gives off a note when it vibrates.

One of the things that causes the vocal cords to vibrate is the pressure of breath released from the lungs when we expire, just as the wind may cause a pair of curtains to flap and give off a sound at an open window. Because the vocal cords are opening and closing many times a second, the expired air is released in a series of infinitesimal puffs; and these puffs of air form a sound wave which carries the tone produced by the vocal cords through the voice tube and out through the mouth.

An increase in the pressure of breath travelling up from the lungs causes the vocal cords to vibrate with greater force, so that they hit each other harder. This produces a louder sound – just as an increase in the force and pressure of a wind would cause a pair of curtains to flap harder and louder at a window. To increase the pressure of the breath travelling up from the lungs through the voice tube, we have to contract the muscles of the chest and abdomen, squeezing the lungs empty with forceful pressure; and this increases the loudness of the voice by causing the vocal cords to hit into each other harder. To decrease the pressure of the breath, we have to ease off the force with which we contract the breathing muscles, squeezing the lungs more gently; and this decreases the loudness of the voice by causing the vocal cords to hit into each other more softly.

The first ingredient of the human voice is therefore loudness, which is perceived on a spectrum from loud to quiet.

Some Psychological Aspects of Loudness

The physical reasons which cause a person to have a loud or quiet voice are connected to the use of the muscles which empty the lungs. But there are often psychological reasons why the muscles are employed in a particular way in the first place.

The quiet voice is often the sound of wisdom; and those with quiet voices may have reached a point where they do not need to make a loud noise, for they rest easily with their insight and are not driven to prove anything. The quiet voice is also equivalent to a soft touch; and some people maintain a voice which touches gently because that is how they wish to be touched. People with quiet voices may be emotionally bruised or sore; and in vocalising softly they may be asking for a tender voice in return to bandage the wounds of their heart. Many people who come into therapy and who find it difficult to produce a loud voice have been assaulted by the insensitive vocal loudness of their parents, partners or other individuals; and they are often frightened of producing a loud voice for fear of becoming like them. In many situations, extreme vocal loudness is associated with negative personality traits such as being 'loudmouthed', impudent, audacious, belligerent and pugnacious. In fact, sounds above 80 decibels are potentially destructive to physical tissue and mental processes. However, it can be a deeply healing experience to access very loud sounds and reclaim the positive side of extreme loudness. For the loud voice is also expressive of elation, excitement, joviality, rapture, rhapsody, celebration and delight; and these qualities can become obscured by an overemphasis on the negative side to loudness. The loud voice is also one way that a person can fill space and claim their territory. The shadow side of this is that loudness also takes space away from others. Producing a loud voice is therefore often difficult for those who find it a struggle to claim their space and their right to a distinctive territory and platform from which to be heard.

There are many people who have no trouble with producing a loud voice and whose therapeutic process is more concerned with uncovering the voice of quietude. Whilst the loud voice halts a listener in their tracks, the quiet voice draws the listener in and is an invitation to intimacy and closeness. Many people develop loud and boisterous voices to mask a fear of such intimacy; and their healing journey often involves dissembling the defence around their vulnerability. Others have loud voices because they have had to shout in order to be heard above the crowd of a large family; and it is often difficult for them to have faith in the belief that they will find satisfaction even if they give voice to their needs quietly. Others have loud voices because they were constantly made to be quiet when they were young and have developed a booming voice as a way of defying this repression.

Like all ingredients, loudness has an almost infinite spectrum of potential psychological meanings which can only be understood accurately in the context of a compassionate and empathic relationship with each individual vocalist. However, the aforementioned ideas provide an impression of some of the more common psychological aspects of loudness.

Practical Method: Developing Loudness

To develop the loudness spectrum of the voice, clients stand comfortably and breathe in and out through the mouth. They then speak a piece of text, vocalising as quietly as possible. Then, they speak the piece of text a second time vocalising at a moderate level of loudness. They then speak the text a third time vocalising as loud as possible. Finally, they speak the text a fourth time and, as they speak, they increase the loudness by degrees moving through the spectrum of loudness from extremely quiet to extremely loud.

Ingredient Two: Pitch

The faster any object vibrates, the higher the note it produces. So the faster the vocal cords vibrate, the higher the pitch of the human voice. To sing the lowest C on the piano, the vocal cords would have to vibrate 32 times per second; to sing the highest C on the piano, the vocal cords would have to vibrate 4186 times per second.

If we wanted to produce a higher note from a vibrating string we would have to tighten it; whilst to lower the note we would have to slacken the string. The same principle applies to the vocal cords. If we tighten and stretch the cords they vibrate at a faster rate and produce a higher pitch; if we slacken them they vibrate more slowly and produce a lower pitch. But the thicker a string is, the more you have to tighten it to produce a high note. This is why the thin strings on a guitar do not have to be tightened as much as the thick strings to produce the same pitch. The same principle applies to the human voice; and because men have thicker vocal cords than women, they have to tighten them more to achieve high notes. Conversely, it is more difficult for women to produce low notes because their vocal cords are thinner. However, the majority of factors which prevent men from singing high and women from singing low are psychological and can be overcome.

The space between two notes is called an interval; and it is the memory of the intervals between notes rather than the notes themselves which enable us to recall a song. When we sing 'Happy Birthday', we can recall the melody because we know the intervals; but the notes themselves are not fixed – we can start the song on any pitch so long as the intervals between all the following notes are correct.

Given that pitch is made up of vibratory frequency, the human voice can obviously sing a vast spectrum of notes by changing the speed of vocal cord vibration. But the European classical Western scale only classes certain frequencies as proper notes. This scale divides the potential range of frequencies into an octave of notes which we can play on the piano. But there are other notes which exist between the keys on the piano which the voice can sing even though there is no string and no hammer for that vibratory frequency on the piano.

Different cultures divide the potential pitch range in different ways. For example, whilst Western music has an octave of eight notes, classical Indian music has a scale of twenty-two notes. What is regarded as a musical note in one place is regarded as redundant in another. But in talking rather than singing, people from all cultures are free from aligning the pitch of their voice with a set scale and the voice rises and falls through the complete range of potential frequencies. This is why singing traditions that originate in the fields and along the railway tracks – where people extend their natural speaking voices into a call – do not suffer from the restrictions of formal music.

With regard to the speaking voice, pitch gives voice its prosody. Without changes in pitch, our voices would speak in monotone. In some languages, the interval between the notes with which syllables are sung actually change the meaning of the word. In Japanese, for example, to rise in pitch at the end of certain words can radically alter the meaning of the word to that imparted when the voice lowers in pitch.

The second ingredient of the human voice is therefore pitch, also referred to as 'note', which is perceived on a spectrum from low to high.

Some Psychological Aspects of Pitch

The height and depth of a voice is dependent on the vibratory speed of the vocal cords, which is in turn dependent on their thickness and the tension of the muscles which tighten and slacken them. But everybody has the capacity to cover an extremely wide pitch range; and the reasons why a person has a particularly high or low voice are primarily psychological.

We tend to raise the pitch of the voice in joy and excitement and people with habitually high voices may seek to reside in the realm of pleasure. But the high voice may also serve as a way of avoiding the sorrowful and somber emotions associated with the deeps.

Like sounds above a certain loudness threshold, sounds produced by extremely high frequencies can be penetrating and destructive. High sounds are usually sensed as being sharp and can be experienced as piercing objects. Some people may develop high voices in order to feel that they have the power to penetrate obstacles, cut through the opposition and forge the way ahead. Other people have extreme difficulty in accessing the high voice because the sense of power which the high voice evokes causes feelings of shame. For those who suffer from a depleted sense of self-worth, accessing the high voice can be extremely empowering. Reaching the high voice can feel as though we have reached new personal heights and achieved a heightened sense of awareness.

High sounds are experienced as being high in space and during a therapeutic process, the vocalist will often reach up with the body as though plucking notes from the air. High sounds instigate feelings of elation and flightiness and for those people who seek to relieve themselves from the depressive monotony of the earth, making high sounds can be extremely liberating. But for those whose tendency is to be ungrounded and unearthed, high sounds can be disorientating and unsettling.

At the other end of the pitch scale is the low voice, which in opera is called bass. This 'bass' voice often expresses the 'base' aspects of our soul which has two dimensions. First, our base is our bedrock, our foundations and the ground upon which our character stands. To access the low voice therefore gives us a sense of deep-rootedness, strength and support. But base also means crude, unrefined, flagrant, obscene and coarse; and vocalising with the low voice enables us to express a certain primeval core of sensation. For those whose healing requires a redeeming of animal instincts and primal passions, the low voice can be very liberating. The low voice feels as though it emerges from deep in the body and making bass sounds can stimulate the sexual organs and stir erotic energy. Many people avoid low sounds as a way of evading their sexuality.

The deep voice is experienced as being low in space and when we vocalise with a bass voice it feels as if we are descending into the deeps physically and emotionally. The low voice can cause us to feel down in the dumps, in the pits, in the doldrums and depressed. Many people have deep voices because their soul resides in the depths of depression; whilst others avoid low sounds so they do not have to confront the morose and depressive aspects of themselves. Our voice descends in sorrow and rises in joy; and many people develop low voices because they have become overwhelmed with sorrow and forgotten the magic of joy.

The low voice sounds as though it emerges from the depths and is therefore associated with depth of integrity, depth of meaning and authority. The high voice can therefore be misread as superficial and lacking in psychological depth. Some people develop low voices in order to preserve a sense of psychological depth whilst others may develop high voices in order to avoid the responsibility which comes with speaking from the deeps.

Like all ingredients, pitch has an almost infinite spectrum of potential psychological meanings which can only be understood accurately in the context of a compassionate and empathic relationship with each individual vocalist. However, the aforementioned ideas provide an impression of some of the more common psychological aspects of pitch.

Practical Method: Developing Pitch

Having explored the spectrum of loudness, clients return to a piece of text and as they speak it they begin ascending and descending in pitch with moderate loudness. When they reach what feels like the top of their pitch range, they try adjusting the loudness to see if this helps them to go higher than they have gone before. They do the same thing when they reach what feels like the bottom of the pitch range. When they have found the level of loudness which enables them to extend the ends of the pitch range, they practise going a little higher and a little lower than they would normally so that in time they extend the range of pitches accessible.

They then speak a piece of text, vocalising in a high pitch range. Then, they speak the piece of text a second time vocalising in a middle pitch range. They then speak the text a third time vocalising in a low pitch range. Finally, they speak the text a fourth time and, as they speak, they move up and down in pitch covering their complete available range.

Ingredient Three: Pitch Fluctuation

When we vocalise, the speed with which the vocal folds vibrate does not remain constant but wavers to some degree. Even if we attempt to sing a single note for a prolonged period of time, for example middle C, the vocal folds will not sustain their opening and closing at an exact and constant 256 times per second. There will be some fluctuation as the vocal cords vibrate a little faster and a little slower in a given unit of time. In Western singing, if the fluctuation is too great, for example fluctuating between 236 and 276 times per second, then the note will sound wobbly and the voice will be judged to be out of tune, particularly if the fluctuation is very slow. But if the fluctuation is minimal – for example between 246 and 266 times per second – and the fluctuation occurs very quickly, then the note will have a quality known as vibrato and the voice will be judged to be classically beautiful. Yet both the revered vibrato and the despised wavering are produced by the same effect. This effect is called pitch fluctuation.

In many indigenous forms of singing the voice is free to fluctuate spontaneously without falling prey to extreme judgements regarding its musical viability. Many of these singing styles originate in the extension of the speaking voice and capitalise on the fact that the speaking voice fluctuates freely in people from all cultures without regard to musical correctness. To draw upon the healing power of the voice we have to suspend our Western judgements and allow the voice to fluctuate freely, just as the soul fluctuates in its wheel of passions.

The third ingredient of the human voice is therefore pitch fluctuation, which is perceived as being fast or slow, great or small.

Some Psychological Aspects of Pitch Fluctuation

In daily life, pitch fluctuation occurs to our voice when we are extremely anxious or nervous; and often the quivering can tingle through the muscles of our whole body. Vocalising with pitch fluctuation can instil feelings of uncertainty, creating the sensation of having an insecure and unstable personality; and those who have a lot of pitch fluctuation in their voice are often of a nervous and insecure disposition. For those whose therapeutic process is concerned with replacing such an unassured persona with confidence and ease, substituting pitch fluctuation with constant tones is extremely assuring. On the other hand, those whose voices lack pitch fluctuation may be holding fast to their security and avoiding the vulnerable and uncertain parts of themselves. For those whose healing requires old patterns to be shaken up and fixed habits to be dislodged, vocalising with pitch fluctuation can provide the earthquake out of which fresh perspectives can grow.

Pitch fluctuation often occurs when we are excited and for those who have lost the elated and tumultuous part of the soul, vocalising with pitch fluctuation can serve to arouse the spirit. But, pitch fluctuation also occurs when we are afraid; and vocalising with pitch fluctuation can evoke feelings of panic and fright. For those whose lives are limited by fear, it is extremely healing to replace pitch fluctuation with constant notes. But for those who want to taste fear again in order to reclaim the sense of forces greater than themselves, vocalising with pitch fluctuation can serve to unnerve the complacent spirit and fill the soul with awe and respect for the unknown.

Like all ingredients, pitch fluctuation has an almost infinite spectrum of potential psychological meanings which can only be understood accurately in the context of a compassionate and empathic relationship with each individual vocalist. However, the aforementioned ideas provide an impression of some of the more common psychological aspects of pitch fluctuation.

Practical Method: Developing Pitch Fluctuation

Now clients have a wide pitch range with which they can begin to speak with varying degrees of loudness, they try to vocalise this range with pitch fluctuation. First, they speak a piece of text, using their complete pitch range, with a very fast fluctuation. Then, they speak the text with a slower pitch fluctuation. As they do this, they vary the level of loudness and continue seeking to go higher and lower in pitch than they have before, allowing themselves to celebrate having three vocal ingredients to experiment with.

Ingredient Four: Register

If you vocalise the lowest note in your pitch range and rise one note at a time up to the highest, you will notice that somewhere in the middle there is a transitional point where a particular change occurs to the quality of the voice. The upper notes will probably seem to have a brighter quality whilst the lower notes will sound darker. The point where this change occurs is called the register break. The two main registers are modal and falsetto. The lower range of notes which sound darker are in modal register and the upper range of notes which sound brighter are in falsetto register. In the Western classical tradition, a female falsetto voice is called 'head register' and her modal voice is called 'chest register'. These terms originate in the antiquated idea that falsetto register generates more vibration in the head whilst the modal register resonates more in the chest; but there is no scientific evidence for this. The term falsetto comes from the Latin for 'false' and calling this quality of voice 'falsetto register' in a male voice and 'head register' in a female voice implies that it is false for a man but not for a woman to vocalise with this quality. Indeed, the association between falsetto and femininity is exaggerated in the pastiche cabaret and pantomime when men use the falsetto register to impersonate the speaking voice of a woman. This is of course unfounded because neither women nor men speak in falsetto, but in modal. But both men and women do use falsetto in their talking voice at times of extreme emotion, such as when we sob or laugh.

In opera, singers are prohibited from exposing the change of register and each singer must use one or the other. The male voices are always sung in modal – with the exception of the male counter tenor – whilst falsetto is reserved for women. But outside of European classical music, in Western contemporary singing and non-Western indigenous styles, both registers are used freely by men and women and are not associated with masculinity or femininity. The register break is particularly exaggerated in the yodelling style of singing often associated with the indigenous music of the Swiss Alps and amongst the North American 'singing cowboys'. Although the higher pitch range of a voice is usually sung in falsetto and the lower pitch range in modal, register is not directly related to pitch because with practice you can vocalise a range of notes in modal and then sing the same range notes again in falsetto.

Because the deliberate exposure of the register break is not allowed in opera, trainees of classical singing learn a technique called blending. This involves ascending and descending the pitch range, gradually blending the qualities of falsetto and modal into a single quality known as a 'blended' register so that the break is eradicated. However, this also eradicates the special emotional magnetism of the register break. To reclaim the full power of the voice, it is necessary to develop both the modal and falsetto registers and allow the voice to move between the two as the mood requires.

The fourth ingredient of the voice is therefore register which is perceived as being either modal, falsetto or blended.

Some Psychological Aspects of Register

A common term for a change in register is a 'break' and indeed as the voice passes from modal to falsetto or vice versa it can feel as though something is breaking. Some people have a constant register break in their daily voice; and often this reveals a deep part of the Self which has been broken and has not healed. Our voice breaks naturally when we are breaking down with emotion; and deep crying is often characterised by a sobbing back and forth between the two registers. But the same register break often occurs when we laugh fully and without restraint. Some people never allow the registers to change, even when they laugh or cry, as a way of avoiding contact with genuine emotion. For those people whose therapeutic journey is concerned with finding access to tumultuous emotions and reactivating the passions of the heart, the register break can be extremely liberating. On the other hand, for those who experience a constant 'breaking' of emotion, replacing the register break with a blended constant quality can be very stabilising and strengthening.

Because, in the West, falsetto is associated more with femininity and modal with masculinity, the vocal registers have a healing power when it comes to sexuality. When a man accesses pure falsetto and a woman accesses pure modal, sexual stereotypes can be overcome and a more holistic sense of gender can be invigorated.

Because the falsetto register is the quality which characterises a child's voice, accessing the falsetto can animate the inner child; and for those who have lost the spirit of youth, this can be very healing. Conversely, for those whose lives are under the constant spell of regression and whose healing journey seeks for an opportunity to mature, the modal voice can be very grounding.

Using the healing potential of the voice involves allowing the voice to break out of one register into another so that we may break out of the fixity of a rigid Self and express our capacity for change and growth. Like all ingredients, register has an almost infinite spectrum of potential psychological meanings which can only be understood accurately in the context of a compassionate and empathic relationship with each individual vocalist. However, the aforementioned ideas provide an impression of some of the more common psychological aspects of register.

Practical Method: Developing Register

Clients start vocalising a note at the bottom of their pitch range and ascend one note at a time, listening for the two notes where the voice changes from modal to falsetto register. They then refind those notes and vocalise them over and over, vocalising on a yodel. Then, having acquired the art of the register break, they practise yodelling in other parts of the pitch range, allowing the voice to create improvised melodies which use modal and falsetto. Finally, they vocalise a range of notes in modal and then practise producing the same range of notes in falsetto.

Clients now speak a piece of text in modal register and then speak the same piece of text again in falsetto register. Then, clients speak the text a third time, allowing the voice to break in and out of the two registers.

Ingredient Five: Harmonic Timbre

The section of the voice tube which runs from the lips to the larynx can change its length and its diameter; and because of the laws of acoustics, the same note produced by the vibration of the vocal cords will resonate with a very different quality if the voice tube is short and narrow to the quality produced when the voice tube is lengthened and dilated.

To understand this, imagine three basic tubes, closed at the bottom but open at the top, constructed to different diameters and different lengths. The first is short and narrow; the second is relatively longer and wider; and the third is much longer and more dilated again. Imagine that we hold a tuning fork vibrating at 256 times per second – which produces middle C – over the top of each tube in turn and listen to the sound of the note echoing or resonating inside the tubes (Figure 3.3). In moving from listening to the sound inside the first tube to the same note echoing or resonating in the second and then the third, we would hear a change of timbre. Perhaps the sound in the first tube would sound 'bright', 'twangy', 'shiny' and 'shimmery'; perhaps the sound resonating in the second tube, by comparison, would sound 'thicker', more 'solemn' or 'fruitier'; and perhaps the sound resonating in the third tube would sound 'full', 'moaning', 'rounded' and 'dark'. Probably, the first tube would sound more comparable to a flute, the second tube would sound more comparable to the clarinet, whilst the sound produced by the third tube would sound more akin to the saxophone; they would all however produce the note C.

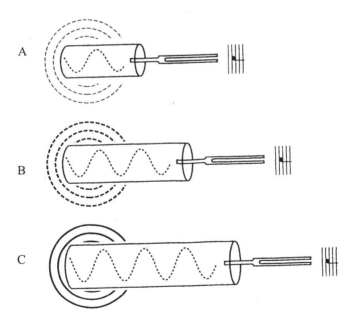

Figure 3.3

With regard to voice production, both the length and the diameter of the voice tube can alter. The diameter of the voice tube can increase by opening the mouth and stretching the throat; and the length of the voice tube can increase by lowering the larynx in the neck. The tube can therefore assume three different configurations comparable to the shapes of the three crude tubes. The first is called flute configuration, whereby the larynx is high in the neck and the tube is quite narrow, such as when we blow a kiss or whistle (Figure 3.4). The second is called clarinet configuration, whereby the larynx is positioned in the middle of the neck and the tube is more dilated, such as when we steam up a pair of glasses (Figure 3.5). The third is called saxophone configuration, whereby the larynx is fully descended in the neck and the tube is dilated to its maximum, such as when we yawn (Figure 3.6).

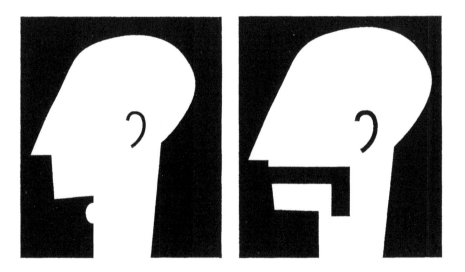

Figure 3.4

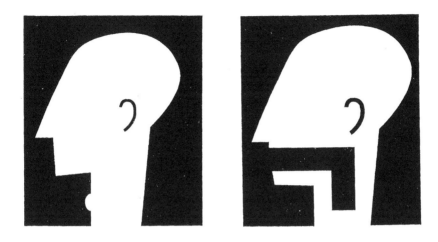

Figure 3.5

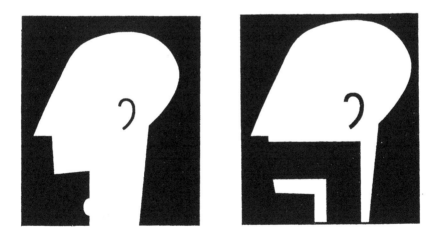

Figure 3.6

If the vibration of the vocal cords is maintained at a constant vibratory frequency, say at 256 times per second, producing middle C, whilst the vocal tract moves from flute configuration through clarinet configuration to saxophone configuration, the effect will be to sing the same note with three very distinct timbres, comparable to that achieved when playing the note C on a tuning fork held above the three separate crude tubes imagined earlier (Figure 3.7). In Voice Movement Therapy, we give the vocal colour produced by a short narrow voice tube the instrumental name flute timbre; we name the vocal colour produced by a medium length and diameter tube clarinet timbre; and we call the vocal colour produced by a fully lengthened and dilated voice tube saxophone timbre.

The fifth ingredient of the human voice is therefore harmonic timbre which can be flute, clarinet or saxophone, depending on the configuration of the voice tube.

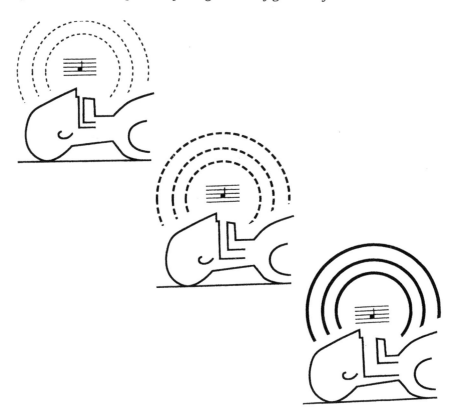

Figure 3.7

Some Psychological Aspects of Harmonic Timbre

The breath emerging from the tube when it is in flute configuration is cool – it is the shape we make with our mouth when we want to cool down hot food by blowing air from the mouth. The sound of the flute timbre can also feel cool, passionless, stoic and frosty. Furthermore, because the flute configuration tube is so narrow, it does not discharge a great deal of acoustic or emotional material and it can sound very reserved and conservative. For those whose therapeutic journey is directed towards learning to preserve more energy and more privacy, such as those who have been depleted and exhausted by their tendency to give too much of themselves, vocalising in flute timbre can be very helpful. But for those seeking to release more of their soul into the world, it is necessary to expand the dimensions of the voice tube. Whilst the flute configuration tends to release a minimum amount of breath and sound, the saxophone configuration releases the entire flood and holds very little back. For those who are seeking to release themselves from the stifling confines of a reserved and retained psyche, vocalising in saxophone timbre can be extremely transforming. Common reasons for expanding the throat to the dimensions of the saxophone configuration are to belch or vomit. Therefore, vocalising with the saxophone timbre can feel as though we are going to bring things up from the stomach. It is, in fact, very rare for someone to actually vomit when vocalising in saxophone timbre; however, it is common for people to initially experience the saxophone timbre as 'sick' and ugly. Although this can be terrifying, it is also very liberating for those whose healing is connected to being released from the pressure of having to be beautiful, sweet and correct.

Another reason for expanding the voice tube dimensions to the maximum is to cry; and vocalising with the saxophone timbre often induces sobbing, which can be very liberating for those who have become separated from their sorrows. On the other hand, for those whose seek to be healed from feeling overwhelmed with the water of their sadness, it is helpful to narrow the voice tube to clarinet or flute.

Between flute and saxophone is the clarinet timbre, which is emblematic of the middle ground. It can narrow to flute or it can expand to saxophone. For those seeking to increase their choices and dexterity, the clarinet configuration is a grail worth pursuing, for it is a platform from which all else is possible.

In Voice Movement Therapy, being able to expand the voice tube dimensions is the single most important part of the physical work. For the expanded tube enables all the other vocal ingredients to be reverberated, amplified and enhanced. Expanding the tube therefore enables people to make the most of themselves, to reveal themselves in all their colours. However, dealing with all the psychological inhibitions which prevent the tube from expanding and the soul from being amplified constitutes one of the most important areas of psychological work. Expanding the tube means expanding the Self; thus it sits at the core of the healing process. I have described at length the physicality and psychology of this process in Volume One of this series *Using Voice and Movement in Therapy* (Newham 1999a).

Like all ingredients, harmonic timbre has an almost infinite spectrum of potential psychological meanings which can only be understood accurately in the context of a compassionate and empathic relationship with each individual vocalist. However, the aforementioned ideas provide an impression of some of the more common psychological aspects of harmonic timbre.

Practical Method: Developing Harmonic Timbre

Clients stand comfortably and breathe in and out through the mouth. They then narrow the voice tube to flute configuration by whistling or blowing cool air as though to lower the temperature of hot food. It is useful for clients to imagine that the voice tube is very narrow and that it extends from the lips down to the indent between the clavicles at the top of the breast bone. They now speak a piece of text, taking the voice up and down the pitch range with varying degrees of loudness in modal and falsetto register, listening to the flute timbre of the voice.

They now expand the dimensions of the voice tube to clarinet configuration, opening the mouth and expanding the throat. It is useful for them to imagine that they are steaming up a window or a pair of spectacles and to feel how the expired breath is now warm. Clients now imagine that the tube is wider and that it extends from the lips down to the centre of the torso at the bottom of the breast bone. They then begin to speak the piece of text a second time, taking the voice up and down the pitch range with varying degrees of loudness in modal and falsetto register, listening to the clarinet timbre of the voice.

They then expand the voice tube to its maximum dimensions, dilating mouth and throat as though yawning and imagine that the tube extends from the lips all the way down into the belly. Clients then speak the text a third time, vocalising up and down the pitch range with varying degrees of loudness in modal and falsetto register, listening to the saxophone timbre of the voice.

Now, they take the text and speak it first in flute timbre then with clarinet timbre and then with saxophone timbre but keeping all the other vocal ingredients constant so that they can hear specifically the three distinct harmonic timbres.

Ingredient Six: Nasality

As the air carries the sound up from the larynx, not all of it passes through the mouth and exits at the lips; some also passes up above the roof of the mouth and through the nasal passages, exiting at the nose. Sound which passes through this tube resonates with a quality which is usually referred to as nasal. In Voice Movement Therapy, we give this nasal quality the instrumental name 'violin' which mixes in with the flute, clarinet or saxophone timbre of the voice.

The more air that passes through the nasal passages, the more nasality or violin the sound of the voice will have; and the quantity of air passing through the passages is controlled by a flap of tissue known as the soft palate. This trap door hangs at the back of the throat and can open and close by degrees. If it is completely closed, then the voice has no violin and sounds lacking in all nasality. If it is completely open, then the voice has a lot of violin and sounds very nasal. Between these two extremes a whole spectrum is possible, like adding or subtracting violins from the string section of an orchestra.

Violin is the quality of voice that children use when they impersonate a Chinese or Japanese person; and though this is a social stereotype, nasality is in fact a tonal colour inherent in a lot of indigenous oriental singing and can be heard in the voices of the Cantonese Opera, the Shanghai Opera and those of the Hút Chéo Folk Theatre of Vietnam.

The sixth ingredient of the voice is therefore nasality or violin which is perceived on a spectrum from minimum to maximum.

Some Psychological Aspects of Nasality

Violin is the quality of voice which people automatically use when impersonating a baby and a very old person. Violin therefore carries with it issues connected to age. People who complain that their voices are too childlike usually have a lot of violin in their voice and by learning to decrease nasal resonance they can experience a new self-image, replacing naivete with maturity.

It is very common for actors to use nasality when playing someone wicked and it is our natural tendency to use violin when we are expressing spite and vindictiveness. For those seeking to get in touch with their malice and animosity, vocalising with violin can be very provocative.

Nasality is an essential component of the speaking voice. In fact, there are certain vowels in the English language, such as 'i' as in 'sit', which can not be adequately communicated without increasing nasality – which is why they are called 'nasal vowels'. In indigenous cultures where the singing style has evolved from speaking and calling, there is often a lot more violin in the voices. Reclaiming the full malleability of the voice means reconnecting to a world voice which can encapsulate the sounds of all nations and all cultures. Accessing violin is therefore a key to sonically empathising with the voices of other lands and can help us get in touch with our multicultural and transpersonal Self.

Acoustically, violin brings to the voice a certain hardness and density, enabling the voice to be projected over greater distances and to be heard above other noise. This is another reason why indigenous singing styles which have originated in the open air and where people had to sing to each other over large distances tend to have a lot of violin in the voices. For those who wish to acquire the ability to project their voice, vocalising with violin is extremely supportive and brings strength and solidity to the sound.

Like all ingredients, violin has an almost infinite spectrum of potential psychological meanings which can only be understood accurately in the context of a compassionate and empathic relationship with each individual vocalist. However, the aforementioned ideas provide an impression of some of the more common psychological aspects of violin.

Practical Method: Developing Nasality

Clients take a note in the middle of their pitch range and vocalise it with moderate loudness without pitch fluctuation in modal register and clarinet timbre. Now, as they produce the note, they add violin by making the sound more nasal. They then practice vocalising this note with a spectrum of violin from minimum to maximum.

Clients now vocalise on another note, again with moderate loudness, without pitch fluctuation and in clarinet timbre, but in falsetto register and practise increasing and decreasing the amount of violin.

Clients now speak a piece of text with lots of violin. They then speak the text a second time with the minimum amount of violin. Then, they speak the text a third time with a moderate amount of violin. Finally, they speak the text a fourth time, varying the amount of violin throughout the speech. When they have acquired control of nasality, they can begin experimenting with different combinations of the other vocal ingredients as they play with the addition and subtraction of violin.

Ingredient Seven: Free Air

When the vocal cords vibrate, they push together momentarily many times per second. But if, during their moment of contact, they do not push tightly together, then breath seeps through the crack. When this happens, the sound of the voice is very breathy. In Voice Movement Therapy such a breathy quality in the tonal colour of a voice is called free air. The more loosely the vocal cords push together, the more free air the voice will have.

The seventh ingredient of the human voice is therefore free air which is generally referred to as the 'breathiness' of a voice and is perceived on a spectrum from minimum to maximum.

Some Psychological Aspects of Free Air

Increasing free air is something which many people do when expressing empathy, gentility and receptivity, whilst voices without any free air usually sound firm. For those people seeking to melt their hard exterior and access their underlying sensitivity, vocalising with maximum free air is ideal. But for those who tend to leave themselves without guard and protection, vocalising with minimum free air can create a greater sense of strength and resilience.

A voice rich in free air is often associated with sexuality; and sexuality is always latently present in the act of singing. The art of singing is, in essence, founded upon the ability to stimulate and arouse the listener with the sumptuous use of the mouth. Some singers have exaggerated the sensual aspect to singing and often use free air to eroticise the tonal colour of their voice. Marilyn Monroe was probably the first to epitomise this style. For those seeking to uncover their buried sexuality, vocalising with free air can be extremely liberating, unleashing the libido in sound.

We also tend to fill the voice with free air when we are exasperated and perplexed; and vocalising with free air can tap into these feelings.

Vocalising with free air is exhausting because the sound absorbs so much breath that you have to replenish the air in the lungs frequently, only to lose it all again in the next sound. This can create a feeling of futility and of 'not getting anywhere'. For people with such a tendency, as well as for those who feel that they lack reserves and who need to lessen their tendency to over-expend, decreasing the amount of free air can be very healing. But for those who feel the tension and pressure of keeping their spirit contained, increasing the amount of free air in the voice can feel extremely releasing.

Like all ingredients, free air has an almost infinite spectrum of potential psychological meanings which can only be understood accurately in the context of a compassionate and empathic relationship with each individual vocalist. However, the aforementioned ideas provide an impression of some of the more common psychological aspects of free air.

Practical Method: Developing Free Air

Clients speak a piece of text in a voice with moderate loudness. They now repeat the text but this time singing it as though they are vocalising on a whisper. As they speak, clients make the sound as breathy as they can, filling the voice with free air. Now, they speak the text a third time and decrease the amount of free air so that the voice is moderately breathy. Finally, they remove the free air completely and speak the text a fourth time with a voice that is firm and solid. Finally, they practice combining varying amounts of free air with all the other vocal ingredients as they speak the text once more.

Ingredient Eight: Attack

The pressure of the breath travelling up from the lungs determines the force with which the vocal cords contact each other during vibration which in turn determines the loudness of the voice. However, the vocal cords also have the capacity to hit each other under the power of their own neuromuscular connections. This means that they can increase or decrease the force of contact. This extra dimension to vocal fold vibration is called attack. Increased attack does not make the voice louder but it gives it a certain stress.

The eighth ingredient of the human voice is therefore attack which gives a voice its stress and is perceived on a spectrum from lesser to greater.

Some Psychological Aspects of Attack

Vocal attack is used when we want to attack our subject with a strength of opinion and certainty and those whose voices are naturally abundant with this quality are often quite strong-minded and strong-willed individuals. We often use increased attack when we are driving our point home with the punctilious and percussive points of our argument. Vocal attack is often used when we are certain of ourselves and those people with a lot of attack in their voices are often those with a sense of self-esteem and sometimes self-righteousness. For those people who have succumbed to this mask at the expense of their vulnerable and uncertain Self, decreasing attack can uncover a tone of greater humility.

Those whose voices lack attack are often dealing with reticence and self-doubt, lacking the necessary belief in themselves with which to attack the world with their voice. For those with a tendency to acquiesce and relinquish their beliefs when intimidated or opposed, vocalising with attack can help to muster a new adversarial spirit and consolidate the ability to hold ground.

Because attack tends to create a percussive dimension, people who naturally use this quality are usually those who think in a linear direction and feel at ease with logic and lists of reasons for and against the decision at hand. Those who lack this quality in their voice, on the other hand, are generally those more at ease with non-linear intuitive thought which meanders and explores issues elliptically. Attack is the rhythmic component to the voice and, for those whose expressions are full of flow but who have lost a sense of tempo in their lives, vocalising with attack can be very grounding. On the other hand, those whose voices have been sequestered by the overbearing demands of time can experience a healing liberation by replacing attack with the soft edges of a gentle tonal colour in their voice.

Like all ingredients, attack has an almost infinite spectrum of potential psychological meanings which can only be understood accurately in the context of a compassionate and empathic relationship with each individual vocalist. However, the aforementioned ideas provide an impression of some of the more common psychological aspects of attack.

Practical Method: Developing Attack

To develop increased attack, clients take a series of vowels preceded by an 'H' and say them quickly and percussively on the expired breath as though they are releasing a series of bullets: Ha, Hi, Ho, He. Then, they sustain the strength of the attack through an extended note on these sounds: Haaaaaaaa, Hiiiiiiii, Hoooooooo, Heeeeeeee. Then, clients speak a piece of text using the increased attack throughout the speech.

Ingredient Nine: Disruption

Sometimes, the two vocal cords do not meet so as to create a flush, smooth edge but instead crash together unevenly with corrugated edges, rubbing into each other and creating friction. When this happens the tonal colour of the voice becomes rough and the pitch becomes discontinuous. In Voice Movement Therapy such a voice is described as possessing disruption. Disrupted sounds also arise when other tissue structures of the larynx vibrate or come into contact with the vocal cords.

The ninth ingredient of the human voice is therefore disruption and is perceived on a spectrum from mild to severe.

Some Psychological Aspects of Disruption

We tend to use disruption when we are extremely angry and when we are scolding someone with a warning; and those with naturally disrupted voices are often host to a backlog of rage. However, the voice also disrupts when we are emotionally disrupted and many people with such voices have been shattered by intense and overwhelming experiences. Conversely, those people who have difficulty vocalising with disruption are often avoiding both their anger and the broken, disrupted and shattered part of themselves. People who cannot access their disrupted voices tend to be stoic and highly attached to the idea of themselves as able and well balanced. For such people, the sound of disruption is too extreme and too threatening, for it promises to overturn the polished persona by sprinkling grit across the smooth surface of the vocal mask. For those seeking to unearth their anger or disturb the perfect grace of their clean-cut person, accessing disruption can be radically transformative.

Like all ingredients, disruption has an almost infinite spectrum of potential psychological meanings which can only be understood accurately in the context of a compassionate and empathic relationship with each individual vocalist. However, the aforementioned ideas provide an impression of some of the more common psychological aspects of disruption.

Practical Method: Developing Disruption

Clients should not practise disruption for longer than a few minutes unless the practitioner is certain that they have been taught a way of creating disrupting sounds which do not threaten the health and longevity of the vocal instrument. As with all of the methods described in this chapter, the practitioner should have mastered the vocal techniques before attempting to impart them to clients. The safest way to get a sense of disruption is to vocalise very quietly in the middle of the pitch range in modal register with very little attack and in saxophone timbre.

Clients begin vocalising on a single note and then start to gently groan as though simmering with fury. As the voice becomes disrupted, they travel up and down the lower part of the pitch range vocalising with disruption. Then, clients speak a piece of text allowing the voice to move in and out of disruption.

Ingredient Ten: Articulation

When we are babies we use the complete palette of articulate shapes available to us as we sculpt vocal sounds with the lips, jaw and tongue. But, when we learn the mother tongue we abandon this range for the narrow spectrum of our spoken language. Only in extreme circumstances, such as speaking in tongues during spiritual ritual or speaking in psychic disarray during mental illness, do we reclaim this spectrum of articulation.

The two units of articulation which are present in all tongues are vowels and consonants. Vowels are open sounds made from a continuous air flow. Consonants are plosive sounds made by interrupting the air flow. In Voice Movement Therapy, articulation does not refer just to the vowels and consonants of a single recognisable linguistic code; it refers to the complete range of articulated structures which can be created by the human vocal instrument. To reclaim the healing voice means returning to the complete palette of sculpted sounds – in effect it means singing in all tongues.

The tenth ingredient of the human voice is therefore articulation which is the sculpting of the vocal sound into vowels and consonants with mouth, lips, tongue and jaw.

Some Psychological Aspects of Articulation

In the early stages of accessing the complete range of the voice, any form of articulation can be restricting, causing the throat to tighten and the voice tube to narrow in preparation for words. But, articulation is also a very liberating ingredient of the human voice because it provides a sense of giving a precise shape to the feeling carried by the voice. For those who find the spoken language of their mother tongue an unfriendly means of communication, singing in a multitude of spontaneous tongues provides a deep level of psychological release as though a new and perfect language has been uncovered.

Practical Method: Developing Articulation

Clients begin by vocalising a long note. They let the voice ascend and descend in pitch and allow the ingredients of the voice to combine spontaneously. Then, they begin to articulate familiar word units: Ta, Go, Sha, Be. As they call out, they start to allow themselves to give shape to word units which are less familiar: Ach, Unf, Tfi, Yin. It is useful for them to imagine that they are touring the world's languages, vocalising excerpts from every tongue that ever was. As they vocalise, they imagine that they are touring the Occident and Orient, the Northern and the Southern hemisphere of the globe and giving voice to the lands which they discover.

The Complete Palette

These ten ingredients make up the palette of tonal colours which can be heard woven into the fabric of every human voice. I have provided a comprehensive demonstration of all the vocal ingredients in the singing and speaking voice on a complete audio course *The Singing Cure* (Newham 1998). To recap, the ten ingredients which make up the human voice are:

> Ingredient One: Loudness, perceived on a spectrum from loud to quiet.
>
> Ingredient Two: Pitch, perceived on a spectrum from low to high.
>
> Ingredient Three: Pitch fluctuation, perceived as being fast or slow, great or small.
>
> Ingredient Four: Register, perceived as either modal, falsetto or blended.
>
> Ingredient Five: Harmonic timbre, which can be flute, clarinet or saxophone.

Ingredient Six: Nasality (violin), perceived on a spectrum from minimum to maximum.

Ingredient Seven: Free air, perceived on a spectrum from minimum to maximum.

Ingredient Eight: Attack, perceived on a spectrum from lesser to greater.

Ingredient Nine: Disruption, perceived on a spectrum from mild to severe.

Ingredient Ten: Articulation, perceived as a sculpting of the voice into vowels and consonants.

A Methodology for Training, Therapy and Analysis

These ten ingredients of vocal expression form the core of the Voice Movement Therapy system which is both an analytic profile for interpreting voices, a psychotherapeutic means by which to investigate the way psychological material is communicated through specific vocal qualities, a training system for developing the expressivity of voices and a physiotherapeutic means by which to release the voice from functional misuse.

Part of the step which I have taken in identifying ten ingredients of vocal expression is to offer a framework within which all voices can be analysed. However, the most significant use of this system is not simply to analyse what one hears, but to enable a single human voice to acquire the dexterity with which to manifest manifold combinations of vocal qualities. When this is achieved, the voice is able to serve both artistic procedures by bringing greater vocal flexibility to the process of vocal expression and is also able to express a greater range of emotional and psychological experience. Voice Movement Therapy is therefore predicated upon a synthesis of analytic, artistic and therapeutic principles.

The set of ten vocal ingredients offers a framework of analysis within which voice production can be analysed intuitively in the absence of objective measuring equipment. For, with training it is possible for an attentive listener to sense the composite combination of the ten ingredients which may be present in a voice at any given time. Those who train in Voice Movement Therapy can therefore learn to hear the voice as comprising a set of vocal tract dimensions and their consequent acoustic timbres known as flute, clarinet and saxophone which can be articulated across a range of pitches, each of which can fluctuate to some degree. These sounds can all be vocalised with degrees of loudness, with a greater or lesser amount of attack and with a spectrum of more or less free air, creating a sound which may be to some degree disrupted and produced in a certain vocal register with a greater or lesser amount of violin.

The various combinations of these ingredients are obviously manifold, each giving specific vocal qualities expressive of particular artistic styles and with particular psychological connotations. Because these vocal ingredients are rooted in the elementary physiological and mechanical operation of the voice, they can be applied with equal efficacy whether analysing vocal expression in a therapeutic setting or vocal styles in an artistic context.

Because the practitioner is approaching the voice subjectively, intuitively drawing upon his or her own responses in the absence of empirical measuring procedures, the Voice Movement Therapy system provides a non-judgemental framework in which to locate such responses. For it is always tempting to analyse the voice by labelling sounds according to emotional, figurative or attitudinal constructs which emanate from the practitioner's own associations. This gives rise to descriptive terms such as 'whiny', 'depressive', 'bubbly', 'childlike', 'aggressive' or 'weak'. In contradistinction to this approach, the provision of measuring devices and the clinical language of allopathic systems describes the voice with terms based in physiological pathology, such as 'hyperkinetic' and 'whispered aphonia'. Whilst the former acknowledges the emotionality and imaginative capacity of the voice, it risks a dangerous disconnection from the mechanics of voice production and can potentially perpetuate a prejudicial reinforcement of vocal stereotyping. The latter, meanwhile, has the advantage of being grounded in an objective understanding of mechanical and physiological voice production and avoids preconceived interpretative conclusions but, on the other hand, relies on scientific procedures and equipment and locates the voice in a language of medicinal pathology which has little to do with the creative and psychological function of vocal expression. The system of voice profile and analysis which I have established offers an opportunity to walk the middle way between these two approaches.

The analytic and interpretative use of the system requires the practitioner to translate associative subjective responses to the vocalist into a profile based on the ingredients. With training, this is possible with some ease because it is these ingredients to which we attend unconsciously when interpreting voices. We may believe someone to be angry because their voice becomes disrupted, the speed of their pitch fluctuation increases, as the sound becomes loud and deep in pitch. We may believe someone is joyous and excited because their voice breaks out of modal into falsetto as it rises in pitch and the quantity of free air increases as the vocal tract lengthens and dilates into saxophone configuration. We may think someone is frightened because their voice has a rapid pitch fluctuation and is very quiet with little attack. We may believe someone to be pessimistic and despondent because their voice is infused with violin and free air within a very small pitch range and is produced with the narrow and shortened vocal tract of flute configuration. This system enables the practitioner to suspend supposition regarding the emotional experience or personality characteristics allegedly expressed and ascertain the component ingredients.

We also listen unconsciously to these ingredients when we hear different performers. Some vocalists utilise free air, others have very disrupted voices. Some types of song or speech are well suited to the expanded saxophone dimensions of the vocal tract, whilst others require the contained nature of the flute configuration. Furthermore, the singing and speaking styles and voice production techniques indigenous to a specific culture tend to favour certain parameter combinations. This component system of intuitive analysis therefore also aims to provide a framework within which various cultural and artistic styles of singing can be located.

The pedagogical use of the system requires the practitioner to teach clients how to attain sufficient malleability of the vocal instrument to be able to combine all vocal ingredients, thereby having at their disposal the broadest possible vocal palette for professional, artistic and personal use. In order to facilitate this in others it is absolutely essential for practitioners to possess such malleability themselves. A significant part of the accredited training programmes in Voice Movement Therapy is therefore focused upon training the student's own voice to manifest a broad range of vocal ingredient combinations. Subsequent to the acquisition of this ability, trainees learn the strategies by which to facilitate maximum vocal expressivity in others.

The process of teaching voice naturally involves investigating both the physical and the psychological reasons for the particular limitations to a client's voice. The application of this system therefore involves a certain therapeutic process on a somatic and psychological level which requires of the practitioner a compassionate, humanitarian and empathic response to the vocal process at all times.

CHAPTER 4

Sounding the Many Selves
Facilitating Personal Transformation through Voice, Mask and Costume

All the World's a Stage

The presence of theatre is woven into the fabric of human expression. For, most of what we do, we do in the presence of others who witness our actions. And, when our actions are witnessed, we may say that we are acting before an audience and that theatre is taking place.

Most people feel that their actions take on a different quality when performed in the company of others. To know that we are being witnessed can often give us the sensation that we are 'on show' and this influences the manner with which we move, speak and behave. The word *audience* comes from the Latin *audio*, meaning 'to hear'; and an audience is essentially and literally a group of people who hear us. The presence of an audience therefore reminds us that we are being heard and consequently draws attention to our voice, which is the acoustic expression of the Self.

An audience is a resonating vessel which amplifies, echoes and reverberates the actor's voice. The manner in which the audience receive sound therefore influences the quality of that sound. That is to say that our voice is influenced by the way we feel we are being heard.

Many people choose to work through an expressive therapy because their difficulties relate specifically to the process of expressing themselves to others. Many people experience extreme difficulty acting authentically before an audience. For such people, life can become an unbearable performance.

In therapy, the therapist plays the role of audience as the client acts the many characters which constitute the *dramatis personae* of the psyche. Therapy is often a theatre for two parties: the actor and the witness. In Voice Movement Therapy, the therapeutic arena is turned into a theatre rehearsal where the client can explore the act of performing to a compassionate witness. And, central to this process is the attempt to empower the client's voice as an expression of their diversity.

Diversity and Rigidity

For many people, their voice becomes acoustically limited to a narrow range of tone and timbre and consequently, the voice communicates the impression of a limited Self to both vocalist and audience.

The material of the voice is sensual and sensory. We hear it through the senses. Frequently we hear the voice as though through the sense of touch. We feel pinched, slapped, compressed, pierced, hammered, stroked, tickled, or shaken by a voice. We hear the voice as though through the sense of taste, listening to the despondent bitterness, the citrus tang of jealousy or the sugary sycophantic sweetness. We hear the colour of a voice, the deep blue of melancholia, the green of envy and the red of retaliation. We may also feel the temperature of a voice, which can be experienced as warm, cool, burning hot or ice cold.

It is not just the listener's senses which are affected by the voice. Often, the presence of a particular vocal quality also affects the way the vocalist perceives his/herself. Our own voice feeds back messages to us through our own ears. Our voice reaffirms who we are, how we are feeling and what we are seeking. The voice serves an important function in maintaining our sense of identity, for the sound of our voice reminds us of who we are, it reinforces our sense of Self. In the same way that our identity is continually reaffirmed by the visual reflection provided by a mirror, so too the sound of our voice enables us to hear reflected an audible expression of our own image. Consequently, changing the quality of voice has the potential to alter both the way others perceive us and the way we perceive ourselves.

As time passes we often become over-identified with a single image of ourselves. We become dominated by the image of our Self as a particular character. We may become stuck in a childlike image, in a dominating and bombastic image, in a kindly and self-effacing image. And all of these self-images find expression through the quality of vocal tones.

Because the echo of the tone of our voice in our own ears is so important in reaffirming our own image, we become caught in a vicious circle. The bitterness or anxiety which we hear in our voice serves only to reinforce the image of ourselves as bitter or anxious. The childlikeness or aggressiveness which we hear in our voice reinforces the idea of our Self as a child or an aggressor. If our psyche becomes so saturated with a single emotional tone, it may become difficult for us to communicate anything else and, without warning, the voice simply lets us down. We may wish to express a particular emotion or image, such as anger or authority; or we may need to instil confidence or calm. But, our voice has become so identified with a particular aspect of ourselves that it cannot move. It is as though the voice has become a rigid mask which we are unable to take off. In fact, the etymology of the English word 'personality' is inextricably linked to the notion of voice and mask. The word 'personality' comes from the Latin *per sona*, which means 'the sound passes through' and was first used to describe the mouthpiece of the mask worn by actors. It then came to denote the character or person which the actor portrayed; eventually it came to mean any person and finally it took on the meaning which it now has for us.

A person with a fixed vocal mask may feel mature but sound childlike; may feel enraged but sound intimidated; may feel saddened but sound unmoved; they seek help but their voice signals self-certainty; they seek warmth and affection, but their voice signals guarded detachment; they seek respect but their voice attracts belittlement. Often this can cause the person some distress, for what people hear on the outside bears no relation to what the person feels on the inside.

Expanding the range of the voice and allowing it to dance freely through all of its colours provides us with an opportunity to step outside the inflexible enclosure of our familiar mask and reanimate the entire kaleidoscope of our personality. Psychologically, this enables us to visit and express those parts of the Self which have hitherto remained in the dark and undercover. By transforming the voice in this way, we can effect changes in the sense of Self. We can provide an opportunity for every individual to hear themselves afresh. Then, when someone can hear themselves as something more than the familiar limited personality with which they have become accustomed, this new refreshed person can be voiced outwardly in the world for others to hear.

The Voice Movement Therapy system described in the previous chapter provides the practical tools with which to transform the Self from a rigid fixity of monocentric identity to a malleable and polycentric wealth of many propensities. By using different combinations of vocal ingredients, we can allow the voice to assume many shades, many colours and many timbres – each one giving acoustic expression to different aspects of the Self. In Voice

Movement Therapy, the skilled practitioner can play a primary role in helping the client release a panoply of inner selves.

Practical Method: The Practitioner as Theatre Director

This is a method by which the professional practitioner helps the client unleash a panoply of characters through an impromptu vocal and physical performance, during which the witnessing therapeutic group help to provide containment by positive and compassionate witnessing.

During the process, the practitioner combines the elements of a number of roles including psychotherapist, masseur, singing teacher, voice coach, theatre director and choreographer. The practitioner's focus is, necessarily, multifaceted during this process, as they manipulate the body, suggest images, enhance the client's breathing pattern and instruct the client in ever fresh ways of combining the set of vocal ingredients. The result is that each client is able to combine an extensive and malleable use of vocal expression with specific combinations of posture and facial expression to palpably formulate a gamut of sub-personalities (see Figures 4.1–4.10).

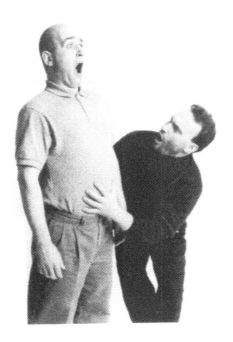

Figure 4.1

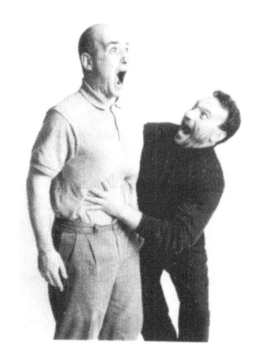

Figure 4.2

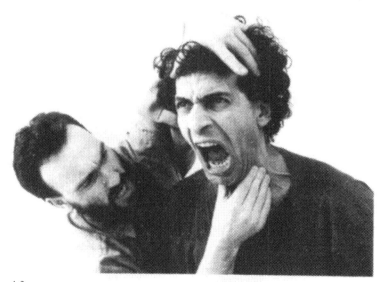

Figure 4.3

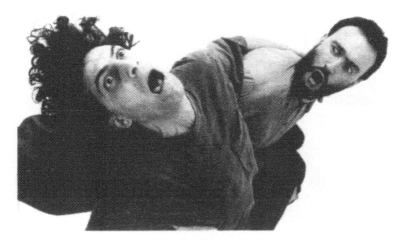

Figure 4.4

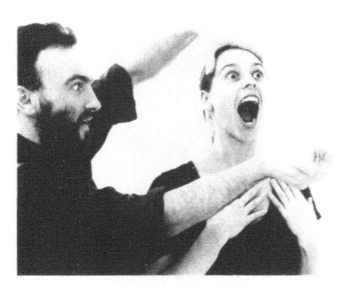

Figure 4.5

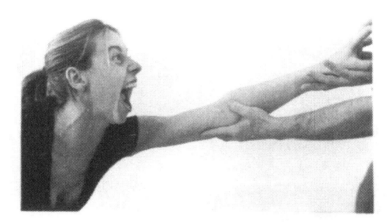

Figure 4.6

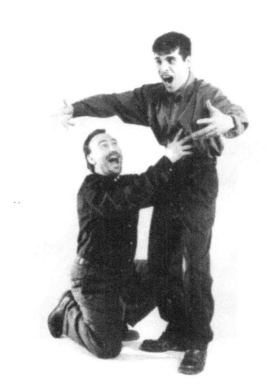

Figure 4.7

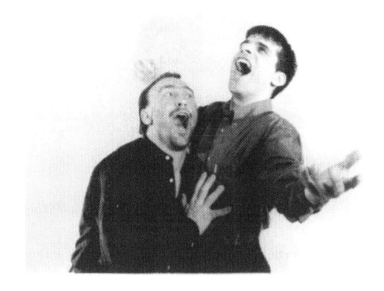

Figure 4.8

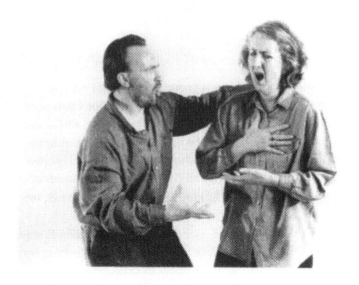

Figure 4.9

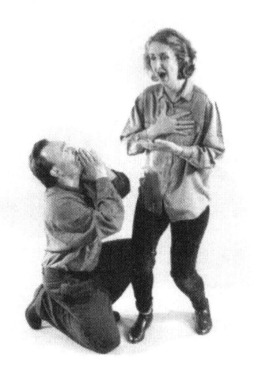

Figure 4.10

For example, imagine the following session. The therapist asks the client to sing, without effort or tension, without demonstration or histrionics. The client sings as herself. The client utters first this note, then that, ascending and descending a scale in which the practitioner can hear or imagines they can hear distinct qualities. For the practitioner, from the perspective of a subjective countertransference, the sound may appear genial and tender with a wispy emission of free air; the higher the pitch the more gentle, soft and unassertive it becomes. It has a girlish frivolity and fragile delicacy to it. The practitioner can see that the client is swaying slightly from side to side and has an ingenuous expression on her face that seems to enhance the innocence of the sound. The practitioner asks the client to exaggerate the swaying as though she were on a swing and to increase the childlike quality of the voice, as though she were only seven years old. The practitioner suggests adding more violin and a mild disruption. The client begins to enter into the embodiment of this image and the practitioner leads the client's pitch up the scale into a higher octave to assist in excavating and refining a sonic and authentic neonatal and infantile image. As the notes begin to get higher, and more difficult to sing, the client contorts the face and clenches her fists which serves to bring to the quality of the sound a degree of ruckus and commotion, as though the baby were having a tantrum. The practitioner asks the client to sing as though the baby were spoilt, irritable, incensed and protesting, and as a result the indignant spectacle becomes more animated and multiphonic. The client opens and closes her fists, stamps on the ground and the practitioner now massages and manoeuvres the neck and back in order to ward off unnecessary tension in the relevant muscle groups. The client continues to vocalise during this massage; her voice increases considerably in volume and height on the pitch scale and whistles through the studio like a siren.

In order to facilitate the sensible experience and personification of the instinctive, natal and primal quality which is emerging, the practitioner asks the client to move into a feline/canine position down on 'all fours' and to allow the voice to move into saxophone timbre as she dances the back and shoulders in an undulating ripple of waves to ensure freedom of corporeal action. The practitioner rhythmically massages the abdominal wall and requests that the client imagines that she howls as though from the abdomen and that the sound resonates inside her belly which is lined with white gold. The sound and personification now glides from the quality of a human baby to a canine quality like that of a howling wolf (Figure 4.11). The practitioner asks the client to imagine that her hackles are up and that she howls a warning and protecting shield of sound around her cubs, which lay curled beneath her belly. The pitch descends and the sound becomes guttural and marauding and echoes as though in a cave. The practitioner asks the client to add a fast pitch fluctuation. In the deeper pitches the sound is wolf-like; in the higher pitches it is feline; in the middle there is an ambiguous animalistic quality, half-wolf, half-cat, like a beast from a beguiling world of creatures concocted from an amalgam of animal instincts.

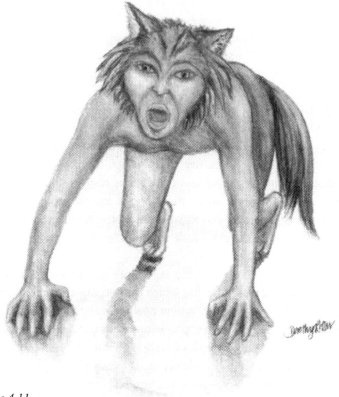

Figure 4.11

The practitioner, having paid passive attention to the client's tendency to open and close the fists during this vocal dance, now asks the client to develop this movement as though she were a creature extending and retracting her claws in preparation for a fight. At the same time she is asked to decrease the volume of the sound and to sing with an alluring, tantalising and ravenous tone, part-lion, part-Siamese kitten, part-wolf. As the client sings, the practitioner continues to suggest tonal images: feline, predatory, devouring, spiteful, provocative, protective. The creature has offspring and is prowling around her young. She spits, with venom, with foreboding and intimidation. Her voice is made of acid, it is caustic, ungracious and scathing.

The client now begins to come up towards a standing posture, and the practitioner suggests the image of a primate, midway between human and animal (Figure 4.12).

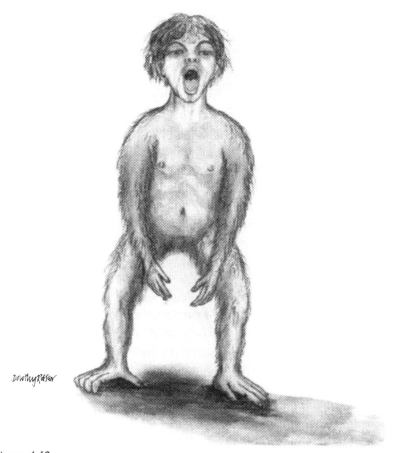

Figure 4.12

The practitioner now influences the melodic direction of the sounds by singing different notes. As the vocal dance assumes a more formal structure, the sounds become humanised without losing their arresting and compelling intensity. The client stands, the voice moves back into flute timbre and the therapist suggests the image of a gigantic Parisian chain-smoking animal-lover with six children who wears a cape and bellows and bawls. The client's voice becomes darkly enfolding which the practitioner amplifies by suggesting a collage of images: a mouth full of caviar, a voice like molasses or like tar, an attitude of belligerent certainty. The voice is that of a prolific and world-famous Parisian lion-tamer.

As the client vocalises, she begins to move her elbows rhythmically, which inspires the practitioner to think of wings. The client now stands on 'tip-toe' and amplifies the wing-like movement of the arms. Her face becomes gaunt as the high pitch combines with low loudness in flute timbre to produce an angelic quality (Figure 4.13).

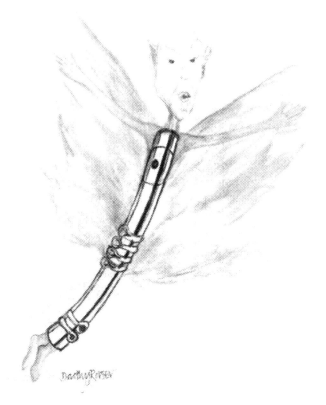

Figure 4.13

The practitioner encourages the client to magnify the choreography of flight and to bring more violin into the voice. Now she becomes a magnificent bird of prey, soaring through the rainforest, parading her kaleidoscopic plumage (Figure 4.14).

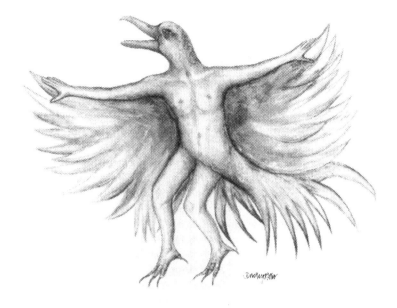

Figure 4.14

As the flight dance exhausts the client, she begins to settle in an erect posture and the bird-like quality subsides to reveal a fresh human sub-personality. The plumage has become a feather cape and hat and the client sings with an air of etiquette and sanctimony (Figure 4.15). A new character emerges and the studio now resonates with the voice of 'Madam Felineou'. The register is falsetto and all the free air has vanished. The client now struts around the studio singing improvised arias on the words 'I am Madam Felineou', like a prima donna. She mimes smoking with a cigarette holder. Her whole face has altered radically from the attitude it expressed at the beginning of the session and any visible or vocal signs of innocence and vulnerability have long since receded. The voice and physicality of the client is dominant, proud and unnerving. The practitioner now asks the client to move from flute timbre to clarinet timbre. As a result the voice takes on a drastic urgency as the client becomes Queen Felineou (Figure 4.16). Now the client is asked to remain in clarinet timbre but to change the register to modal and as she does this, the characterisation becomes masculinised as the client sings in a bombastic baritone, playing with different intensities of vibrato as she sings 'I am King Felineou' (Figure 4.17).

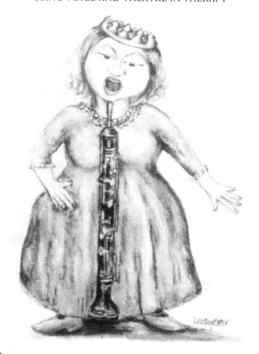

Figure 4.15

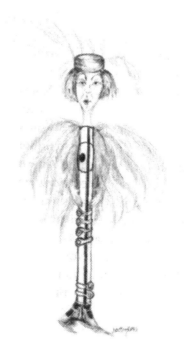

Figure 4.16

The practitioner now asks the client to magnify and inflate the masculinity and to personify the image of a warrior. The client mimes the carrying of a spear and the voice now takes on a hot-blooded, ambitious and barbarous tone (Figure 4.18). The practitioner encourages this transformation by suggesting tonal images: wild man of the forest, revengeful war cry, leading the warriors into battle, rounding up a tribal mass of agitated protesters. The client's voice and body is now involved in an opera of blood curdling melody as though the studio were full with an army of rebels.

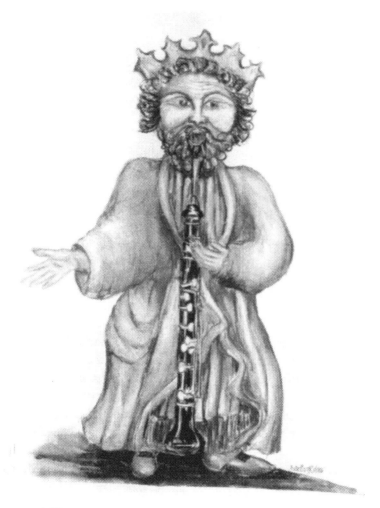

Figure 4.17

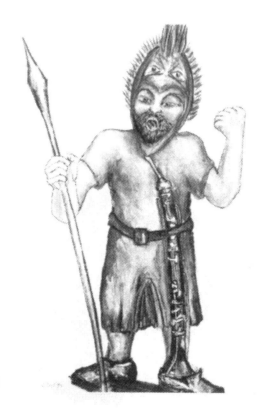

Figure 4.18

The client is becoming tired, and the practitioner slows down the pace through gentle instruction. The dead lay scattered and the wild woman now feels sorrow for the victims. The voice returns to a higher pitch and whimpers. The practitioner suggests tonal images: pangs of regret, mourning and melancholy; a prayer for the dying; and a contemplative chant on the futility of war. The practitioner suggests that the client allow free air to re-enter the voice. The client now stands swaying, as she was at the beginning of the session and the practitioner asks her to blend in different aspects of the acoustic journey into a single tone. The irritable child, the vulnerable kitten, the howling wolf, the wild woman of the forest, Madam Felineou and the unbridled warrior become less separate and distinct voices and more aspects audible in a single tone. The voice sounds and feels to practitioner and client that it belongs to her. But it is multifaceted, embracing and containing a spectrum of images any one or combination of which could emerge as the dominant factor at any time.

The process of transformation from this wolf image to the image of Madam Felineou is a slow one, in which every stage of the transformation from the howling wolf to the meowing cat-woman is fleshed out, filled in, satiated and made specific through precise alterations in acoustic quality and kinetic gesture. From baby to wolf, from wolf to wolf-cat, from wolf-cat to primate, from primate to flying angel, from flying angel to soaring bird, from soaring bird to Madam Felineou and Queen Felineou, then from Queen to King and from King to Warrior. But all of this has nothing to do with the generalised mimicry of putting on different voices, such as that heard in pastiche cabaret, and when the vocalist succumbs to the superficial option of mimicry, not only the attuned practitioner and the client but anyone else who may be present in a group session can hear it.

The professional practitioner must help to amplify, embellish, fertilise, enrich and refine the timbral qualities which are present in the voice but must not generalise and abstract all detail; they must remain attentive to specifics, which requires acute listening. Furthermore, the practitioner must not be influenced by their own modalities or imagistic preoccupations. They must not trespass eagerly forward according to their own tastes. They must not adorn and decorate through suggestions which emanate from the prejudice of their own ears. The images supplied by the practitioner must originate in the acoustic information supplied by the client and must be amplified to embody images of a genuine significance, culturally and personally, and not to reflect the widespread social stereotypes to which modern men and women have become prey. This requires of the practitioner an intimate and well-tested exploration of his or her own subjective reactions, that is their countertransference.

The advantage of this method is that an able practitioner can intervene and enable the client to avoid employing unhealthy methods of voice production and avoid repeating patterns of vocalisation which compound restriction and inhibition. The disadvantage of this method is that the client is steered directively and is not completely free to experience the contours of the psyche uninfluenced by the witness. This is why Voice Movement Therapy provides a number of practical methods by which the client can explore the psyche free of the practitioner's interventions.

Practical Method: The Inner Cast

The client is asked to consider the way that they are composed of many different characters, personalities or figures which act their various roles at different moments in the course of a day or a month or a year. Usually, clients are asked to conceive of somewhere between four and twelve figures.

The client is asked to name each of these figures in some way and then to produce a short monologue for each character written in the first person. The monologue should introduce the character and describe their relationship to the client. Clients need to be given time to pursue this task, usually about one to two weeks between therapeutic sessions.

The client then reads each monologue to the practitioner and, in the case of group work, to the therapeutic group.

Case Study: Richard

Don't Bring Me Down

Richard, whom I first introduced in *Using Voice and Song in Therapy* (Newham 1999b), was one of a few who had survived an aeroplane crash. Though he had remarkably and miraculously not sustained any serious physical injury, the event had severe consequences regarding his mental and emotional life.

His symptoms included insomnia, nightmares, periods of extreme depression, suicidal fantasies and panic attacks. Before the accident, Richard had been an outspoken person with a loud and resonant voice. Now, his speaking voice was almost a whisper and he felt nervous when called upon to speak up for himself. Richard had come into therapy because he wanted to refind both his singing voice, in order that he could rejoin a choir, and his speaking voice, so that he could 'begin to put his life back together'. Since the accident he had felt 'stuck' and 'entrenched' and was desperate to refind some 'vitality' and 'motivation'.

When Richard was asked to pursue this exercise he met with some resistance which, when analysed, revealed itself to be rooted in his fear that he would not be able to 'come up with any sub-personalities'. My response was to ask him which part of himself or which figure it was that was afraid of this emptiness. He replied: 'I guess it's the downer in me, the bit of me that immediately thinks whatever is to come my way is going to get me down'. I suggested to Richard that this was probably his first figure and that he should start with that one. He did not seem happy or encouraged but said he would 'do his best'.

Next session, Richard returned to the group with seven figures which he had named as follows: The Downer, The Stubborn, The Coward, The Stoic, The Pioneer, The Singer, The Mute.

The following are brief excerpts from the monologues which Richard read.

THE DOWNER

I am The Downer and I am always down, even when the sun is shining and everybody else seems to agree that the day is going to be bright, I still look grey and feel blue. My relationship to Richard is that I stop him having any fun and remind him that very serious things have happened to him and might happen to him again, so he better be prepared and not let slip and have any fun.

THE STUBBORN

I am The Stubborn and I dig my heels in and wont let Richard move forward if I feel it cannot be done; and as I think most things cannot be done, Richard doesn't move forward very much these days.

THE COWARD

I am The Coward and I am very very afraid. I make Richard feel like a little child who is scared to come out from under the bed clothes. I make it hard for Richard to get out of bed in the morning and when he is up and about, I make him feel very small.

THE STOIC

I am The Stoic and I push Richard forward even when The Downer, The Stubborn and The Coward want to hold back. I give Richard support and strength and enable him to do things that he would rather shy away from. I make Richard pull himself together when he is falling apart at the seams and I make him put on a brave face so others don't see how foolish he is.

THE PIONEER

I am The Pioneer and I am pushed to the back and trampled on by The Coward who is stronger than me. So I don't get a chance to help Richard very much. But when I do, I enable him to go places he would not normally go and do things he would not normally do. I am not afraid to experiment with new ideas and when I get a chance, I help Richard discover the excitement of life.

THE SINGER

I am The Singer and I give Richard a voice which makes him feel warm and alive. I provide Richard with a key to his heart and I help him feel his deepest emotions.

THE MUTE

I am The Mute and I say nothing. I keep quiet and hold everything in so that Richard does not blurt out something stupid or make himself sound like a fool.

Richard read each monologue from the page with a task-like demeanour and without visible signs of any particular or extreme emotion. When he had finished, however, he smiled with a look of accomplishment. Richard had moved from thinking that he could not do the exercise to producing some very insightful work.

Client's Account: Richard

Overturning the Inner Government

I struggled hard with doing this exercise because I really thought I could not do it; and the excitement expressed by others in the group at doing it just made be more stubborn that I was not going to do it and more afraid that I could not do it.

However, when the group leader pointed out that in some way my emotional reactions to doing the exercise may provide me with the very foundations of my inner figures, I was able to see things in a new way. My first two figures, The Downer and The Stubborn were born out of me feeling that the exercise was going to get me down, and my stubborn feelings of determination that I was therefore not going to do the exercise.

Then I began to feel like a bit of a coward, especially as many others in the group seemed to be braving the task with open arms. So my next figure became The Coward because I do feel I am often cowardly when it comes to stretching myself. By this point, I decided that I would go on and do my best, which reminded me of my stoic trait which I got from my father. He rarely showed any emotion, especially in the face of suffering, but went on with a stiff upper lip. So my next figure became The Stoic. However, having been set to thinking about my father, I started to realise that I had also inherited from him an incredibly pioneering spirit. In fact, before the accident, I had been very novel and imaginative in breaking new ground in my profession. So, I stopped giving myself such a hard time and made my next figure The Pioneer. The last two figures, The Singer and The Mute, came to me a few days later when I was considering why I was pursuing this therapy in the first place. Having created seven inner figures, I actually felt quite pleased and found the task of writing the monologues very helpful.

Writing the monologues enabled me to see a sort of mechanism that I think is at work in me. It is as though I am governed by the board of seven advisers who have known each other for a long time and who are sort of stuck in their ways. They all think that they have my best interests at heart, yet if they had been allowed to have their way, I would probably not have done the exercise. But for me, the most liberating part of the exercise was that I felt that I was diagnosing and describing myself rather than have a therapist do it for me. And, most importantly, I felt that I needed to uncover some other figures to counteract the influence of the first seven on my life.

Working with sub-personalities seemed to make the inner work that I needed to do a creative and – dare I say it – quite simple task. It became clear that what I needed to do was to dig deep into myself and rescue some other figures. I needed to effect an inner revolution where the crusty and complacent Board of Seven Governors were joined by some fresh blood. I needed to give some other parts of me a voice.

Case Study: Teri

The Brat and Baby Blue

Teri, whom I first introduced in *Using Voice and Song in Therapy* (Newham 1999b), was in the same therapeutic group as Richard for a period of time. She came into therapy because she felt her voice was too high in pitch, too 'breathy' and too 'childlike'. She described herself as feeling 'small' and felt that people did not take her seriously. Teri had chosen to work through Voice Movement Therapy in the hope that it might enable her to lower the pitch of her voice and to sound 'more mature', and at the same time help her to 'grow' and 'mature' in herself.

Teri's parents had separated when she was eight years old and she had lived permanently with her father, visiting her mother for one day, twice a month. Her mother had been an alcoholic as well as suffering from intermittent mental illness. Teri had one brother, four years her senior, who went away to college when he was sixteen. Teri had therefore lived alone with her father from the age of twelve until she left home at eighteen. Teri loved her father; she almost idolised him. He had protected her, cherished her, doted on her every smile, succumbed to her every wish and provided for her every need – so long as she remained his little girl. When she reached adolescence and began to want the freedom to explore the world beyond the exclusivity of the paternal dotage, her father had not been so good at letting her go as he had been at keeping her near. Teri's father died a few years before she came into therapy, in fact it had been one of the events which prompted her to seek some therapeutic help.

Teri had not only been overprotected, mollycoddled and girlified by a father who wanted his daughter to remain his princess and replace the sweet wife he had lost to wild abandon. Teri had also been discouraged from expressing any kind of voracious or intemperate feelings because it reminded her father too much of Teri's mother. In fact, Teri recalled a number of times when her father had told her that if she continued to 'behave that way' she would 'end up' like her mother. In many ways, Teri kept herself from growing up and finding the voice of a woman because her first and most potent experience of a woman was her mother who had been presented as crazy, out of control and incapable. Teri did not want to become her mother, so she played into the hands of her father and remained a little girl and from here she went into the lap of her boyfriend who was twelve years older than her and who encouraged the same childlike parts of her.

Unlike Richard, Teri said that she enjoyed doing this work and that it lifted her spirits. She felt that it was exactly what she needed to help her uncover more of her adult self. Her figures were named: Baby Blue, Big Brat, Daddy's Girl, Mad Mom, Mousy Milly, Pleasing Polly and Seething Susie. She introduced each monologue with the name of the figure and one sentence which encapsulated the relationship between the figure and Teri. Then she proceeded to read the monologues which all had the feel of a nursery rhyme. The following are excerpts from the monologues which she read.

BABY BLUE

My name is Baby Blue and I make sure that men find Teri sexy and want to possess her.

My name is Baby Blue and I can do it for you. Whatever your heart's desire, I can light your fire. I'll make your juices flow and your member grow, cos I am Baby Blue and I can do it for you.

BIG BRAT

My name is Big Brat and I make sure Teri gets what she wants.

My name is Big Brat and I want what I want when I want it and I usually get it. So give me, give me, give me, or I'll scream and scream and scream. You know its best to keep me quiet so fill me up with what I want and don't make me ask again.

DADDY'S GIRL

My name is Daddy's Girl and I make sure that Teri remembers that her daddy is the best man and that she will always be a little girl.

I am Daddy's Girl and I belong to no other. I loved my daddy very much but I have to make do with mother. Daddy's gone but loves me so and looks down on me from heaven. Sometimes I wish that I could die so I could hold his hand. For life without daddy seems so sad and ever so ever so bland.

MAD MOM

I am Mad Mom and I remind Teri that if she lets herself feel too much too intensely she will go mad like her mother

I am Mad Mom and I am as mad as a thumb in a plumb or a snowflake sandwich or a five-legged artichoke on wheels.

MOUSY MILLY

My name is Mousy Milly and I make sure that Teri doesn't get too serious or grown up so that people will not ask too much of her so that she can continue to play.

My name is Mousy Milly and generally I am very silly. I squeak and giggle and scratch and wriggle and my dresses are usually quite frilly.

PLEASING POLLY

My name is Pleasing Polly and I aim to get Teri to please people by doing whatever they want so that she can feel useful and loved.

My name is Polly and I like to please. I cook and clean and scrub and wash and my work never seams to cease. But if it makes you smile then it makes me feel good; for it stops me feeling useless and hopeless and spoilt. So whatever it is you want, just give me a call and I will come running and please you in a flash.

SEETHING SUSIE

I am Seething Susie and I make sure Teri doesn't forget her true feelings which she is often afraid to show.

I am Seething Susie and I seethe and fume and smoulder. I am full of hate for most of those around me. I hate Big Brat because she has to behave like a baby to get what she wants and this makes her look stupid. I hate Daddy's Girl because her daddy is dead and she won't let go and this makes her look stupid. I hate Mousy Milly because she is silly and I hate Pleasing Polly because she behaves like a slave. The only one I like is Baby Blue – she's orgasmic.

Client's Account: Teri

Growing Up

I found the work both very enjoyable and at the same time shocking and a bit of a revelation. The most striking thing was how most of my figures were like kids in some way – apart from Seething Susie. During the whole process of writing the monologues I felt like a kid at school doodling. It did not feel like I was doing serious therapy; somehow I was just playing around. But then I realised that this reflected exactly how I feel in the world most of the time. I feel like I am a kid in a playground and everyone else is in the grown up world. This makes me feel quite safe and protected but at the same time makes me feel small and incapable.

I realised too that my figures were very much geared to either getting what I want from others or giving others what they need. I didn't find any figures which just had their own personality. When I had finished creating them, I did not like them very much. I felt they kept me locked into a certain way of being, and from these feelings of hate towards my own figures I created Seething Susie. I think Seething Susie is the most important figure for me at the moment.

Practical Method: Differentiating the Voices

For the next stage, clients are asked to experiment with their voices, finding a specific combination of ingredients for each sub-personality which brings the particular characteristics of the sub-personality into sharper focus. Using the Voice Movement Therapy system, clients are encouraged to try out different vocal qualities for each sub-personality until they find a vocal quality for each which feels suitable. Finding the diversity of voices usually influences the entirety of the client's presence, and there is a visible alteration in the posture, facial expression and dramatic attitude each time a new vocal sub-personality is crafted. In this way, the voice acts as a catalyst for complete psychosomatic transformation. The client then practises delivering each monologue in the particular chosen vocal combination of ingredients, using the Voice Movement Therapy system. The monologues are then presented again.

Case Study: Richard

Escaping the Monotony

Richard seemed to have great fun experimenting with his voice and fleshing out his sub-personalities with specific vocal qualities. The combination of vocal ingredients which he used for each character were:

- The Downer: quiet, low pitch, saxophone timbre, modal register.
- The Stubborn: medium loudness, medium pitch, clarinet timbre, modal register, attack.
- The Coward: quiet, high pitch, flute timbre, falsetto register, free air.
- The Stoic: quiet, low pitch, clarinet timbre, modal register, attack, violin.
- The Pioneer: loud, medium pitch, saxophone timbre, modal register, violin.
- The Singer: loud, high pitch, clarinet timbre, falsetto register, pitch fluctuation.
- The Mute: quiet, medium pitch, flute timbre, free air, disruption.

Richard's presentation of his monologues was radically different this time. For, the voices gave each sub-personality such distinctive contours that it became possible to see the rich diversity beneath Richard's usually nonexpressive manner. Richard was someone who felt stuck and sounded stuck; there was a fatigue and despondency to his voice and choreography. However, in the presentation of his monologues, a fresh life-force seemed to come shining through, as though he had escaped the monotony of his depressive tendencies.

Client's Account: Richard

Feeling the Vibrations

> Giving my sub-personalities specific voices shocked me. When I was presenting the monologues in pretty much the same quality of voice, they were not really part of me – they were ideas. But as soon as I started using different voices to articulate the sub-personalities, there was no escape from the fact that these people were part of me. They emerged from inside me. I could feel them vibrating inside me and then they came out of my mouth in sound. For the first time I could feel how these figures influence the way I give voice to myself in the world. Because, although in daily life I do not change my voice as much as I did in the presentation, nonetheless, the same changes are present in a subtle way. I am these people and these people are me.

Case Study: Teri

Changing Tune, Changing Face

This process of differentiating the voices of the sub-personalities presented a great challenge to Teri, because part of her reason for undertaking Voice Movement Therapy was her sensation of having a very limited vocal range. To help Teri, I gave some focused technical instruction which enabled her to access the vocal ingredients which she found most foreign. She was then able to connect the vocal techniques to the psychological investigation of her many selves and locate the appropriate voice for the right character. Her vocal characteristics for each sub-personality were:

- Baby Blue: quiet, middle pitch, clarinet timbre, modal register.
- Big Brat: loud, high pitch, flute timbre, falsetto register, attack, violin.
- Daddy's Girl: medium loudness, high pitch, saxophone timbre, falsetto register, free air.

- Mad Mom: loud, high pitch, saxophone timbre, falsetto register, pitch fluctuation, attack, violin.

- Mousy Milly: quiet, medium pitch, flute timbre, falsetto register, free air, violin.

- Pleasing Polly: medium loudness, medium pitch, clarinet timbre, modal register, attack.

- Seething Susie: loud, low pitch, clarinet timbre, modal register, attack, disruption.

Hearing Teri present each monologue again with this range of vocal qualities was quite spectacular. As she moved from one sub-personality and set of vocal ingredients to the next, her entire demeanour changed, including her physical stance and her facial expressions. It was clear that she had found something important.

Client's Account: Teri

Feeling Big at Last

Using the vocal ingredients to make each character different was incredibly uplifting for me. Because, although I was not fond of all my characters, I found that I could produce so many different kinds of vocal sounds and this made me feel big and able, as though there was a lot more to me than even I had thought.

I realised that my feelings of being small were also feelings of being stuck in one place, in one picture of myself. To feel that I could be many people and have many voices made me feel fuller, richer and that I was big in a way that I hadn't thought of. Before doing the sub-personalities with the voices, I had thought that I needed to change my little voice for a big voice and learn to be more domineering. But actually, I realised that what I really need is to allow all the different parts of me to be voiced. That is the bigness that I want.

But the biggest shock for me was hearing myself do the voice for Seething Susie: the low, loud disrupted sound was a voice I have never made before and would never have imagined that I could produce. It made me feel my power and my rage – I could feel the sound make my whole body shake.

I always knew that I had a fire in my belly, but I thought that the flame had just gone out. But using the combination of loudness, low pitch, clarinet timbre, modal register, attack and disruption made me feel alive and burning. I think it was the first time I had felt the fire in me rekindled for a long time.

Practical Method: Costuming the Figures

Clients are now asked to find costumes for each sub-personality. Clients are encouraged to consider using accessories including hats, gloves, umbrellas, canes, fans, jewellery and bags as well as clothing. Again, clients need to be given time for this task, usually a minimum of a week. This enables the process to work upon the client therapeutically and gives space within which discoveries can be integrated.

On returning to the therapeutic session, clients revisit the stage and present each figure, delivering the monologue with the previously selected combination of vocal qualities, but this time in costume. Changing behind the screen they appear as each character in turn. Clients are asked to spend a little time walking, sitting and standing allowing the costume to influence their style of motion and mannerisms. This not only refines the literal and metaphorical 'voice' of the sub-personality but also adds to the physical, facial and attitudinal embodiment of each one.

Practical Method: Masking the Figures

Having presented their costumed figures, clients are now asked to make a mask for each sub-personality. Clients are encouraged to use any materials and to consider that the purpose of the mask is to give each of their figures a definite face. On returning to the therapeutic session, clients revisit the stage and present each figure again in costume and mask.

Changing behind the screen they appear as each character in turn. Clients are asked to spend a little time walking, sitting and standing allowing the costume to influence their style of motion and mannerisms. They then speak excerpts from their monologues again in full costume and mask, using the Voice Movement Therapy system of vocal ingredients to continue differentiating the vocal characteristics of each sub-personality.

Practical Method: Relating with the Figures

For the final stage of this journey through the many selves, members of the group are asked to form groups of two, three or four. A stage is then set up which has a boundaried performance platform and a screen behind which clients can disappear to get changed.

In the small groups, clients enact an improvisation where the sub-personalities of each client interact with the sub-personalities of the others in the small group. At any point a client may leave the stage and disappear from the audience's view by going behind the screen. They then reappear dressed and masked as a different figure.

Client's Account: Richard

The Sexy Pioneer

> I was in a group with Teri and found it quite a transformational experience because I found that my feelings towards Teri completely changed depending upon which sub-personality we were both presenting. With some combinations, like her Pleasing Polly and my Stubborn personality, it was impossible to make anything happen because the more she tried to please me the more stubborn I became that I did not want to be pleased. But other combinations were electric and uncovered parts of me which I would not normally show.
>
> For example, the combination of Teri's Baby Blue and my Pioneer was very exciting. I do not normally experience myself as a sexual person and do not feel that women are attracted to me. But because Teri was so persistent – that was the nature of her Baby Blue character – I had no choice but to respond. So my pioneering sub-personality led me into flirting and courting with ease – something I could not have imagined doing.
>
> But this only happened because Teri's Seething Susie had been so aggressive towards my Coward sub-personality that I just could not take any more – this was when I changed into my Pioneer.

Client's Account: Teri

Relying on Sex

> I have to admit that when I was presenting my Seething Susie sub-personality and I saw Richard presenting his Coward, I got so angry. I remember yelling at him: 'Come on, be a man – what are you afraid of'. At first, the more seething I was, the more cowardly he became. I did not know where this vitriolic behaviour was coming from, but I just kept on at him, wanting him to give up his cowardice.
>
> Then, I think Richard snapped, because he changed into his Pioneer sub-personality which completely threw me. There was something about

this character which, rather than making me seethe, made me feel like I wanted to go forth and be pioneering with him. So I changed into my Baby Blue sub-personality and we began this kind of erotic playfulness.

Afterwards, on reflection, I realised how the only way I feel I can be equal to a man and be with a man as an adult is through being sexual. I did not have a sub-personality which I could bring forward that would have enabled me to relate to Richard's Pioneer without an overt sexual component. I realised that this was a part of myself that I needed to find.

Expanding the Self

Having explored the use of sub-personalities through text, voice, costume and mask to this point, clients may go on deepening the work by uncovering new personalities and bringing them into interaction with the sub-personalities of others in the group. The work is almost endless, and it is the role of the practitioner to help the clients challenge themselves by taking the risk of bringing previously unexpressed parts of themselves onto the therapeutic stage where they can be reshaped and reinvented through the process of improvisation with others. The voice is crucial in this process, for it is through the dedication to giving each sub-personality a specific acoustic form that they move from the realm of idea to the realm of embodied sensation.

CHAPTER 5

The Theatre of Family Life
Tracing the Personal Origins of Vocal Identity

The History of Selves

During the exploration of the many selves, as described in the previous chapter, it is very common for clients to recognise that some of their sub-personalities are directly descendent from aspects of their parents. It is as though some of the parents' qualities have been absorbed by the client and have constellated into distinct selves which emerge in a variety of ways, including through vocal expression. In addition, clients often realise that their own personality and their own voice has developed in response to the family constellation and the implicit demands of the parents. Indeed, the family circumstances constitute the single most influential factor in the shaping of a client's voice.

The Amniotic Orchestra

The gestating babe-to-be is suspended in the amniotic haven of the womb. It is enclosed and enwrapped in a warm, wet pocket of darkness where it rehearses the dance of life, extending the spine, gyrating the limbs, marking out the movements of breathing, opening and closing the mouth, cultivating the art of yawning, acquiring the technique of swallowing and practising the template of movements that it will need at birth and beyond. This gestation and incubation takes place in a sanctuary of sound without light. For the growing babe hears but does not see.

The gestating foetus is like a giant ear and is highly sensitive to the orchestra of acoustic movements which permeate the abdominal wall and stir the amniotic fluid with a vibration of sound waves. The sonorous ambience of the mother's environment creates an auditory impression of the world for the growing babe; and these sounds encompass and envelop the baby completely. Sound passes through the wall of the womb and ripples the amniotic fluid, creating sound waves which encircle the baby as the ripples on a pond surround a pebble. The baby feels sound bodily as though it were touching the entire surface of the skin. The sounds which erupt and resound in the mother's world are echoed in the waters of the womb and etched upon the baby's skin like a calligraphy of virgin experience.

The growing foetus is so sensitive to sound that a newly born baby can recognise the specific musical contours of the mother tongue. A baby born to a French-speaking mother will lose interest in suckling and express disturbance if the mother starts speaking in Russian, but will resume feeding with pleasure when the mother resumes speaking in French. The reverse is true for a baby born to a Russian-speaking mother who will feed enthusiastically whilst the mother speaks in Russian but will disengage and agitate if the mother starts speaking in French. The ears of the gestating foetus are hugely sensitive, not only to the contours of the language spoken on the other side of the abdominal wall, but also to emotional expressions and atmospheres. A mother experiencing depression, anxiety or insecurity influences the growing babe. An environment aloud with sounds of anger and conflict is impressed upon the growing infant. When the baby is born, it already brings with it a certain intra-uterine aural history of the world – a world which it sees for the first time but has heard and felt before.

The newborn baby passes into this world already carrying a history of nine months; and most of this history has been acquired through the medium of sound. The star of this constant opera is the mother, to whom the growing babe listens attentively from within the auditorium of the womb and whose voice resounds like a diva for forty weeks. When the baby emerges into the light of life, it does not meet the mother for the first time, for her voice is known. The mother's voice is woven into the fabric of the baby's psyche and continues to be a highly significant source of sensation and experience.

In the womb, the babe can hear but cannot respond. In gestation we are mute and unheard. But birth releases the babe from silence and the cry of the human voice is the first mark which the newborn infant makes upon the world. The young infant does not speak with words but paints with sounds, relying on the choreographic dance of the body and the melodic singing of the voice to express the nuance and cadence of feeling and sensation. The mother listens to her baby's songs and replies with her own improvised arias; and the mother's voice can be as nourishing to the baby as her milk. Babies suckle more vigorously when accompanied by the sound of their mother's voice; but when this is replaced with another voice, with recorded sounds or with instrumental music, the baby loses interest in feeding.

Suckling and Singing

The newly born infant experiences one of its first and most primary instincts in the stomach; and its hunger is expressed through the emission of sound through the mouth. The baby feels an emptiness, a hollow yearning for nourishment and it is this instinct to feed which rises up from the belly and out through the voice tube in the form of a hunger cry, an imploring for food. Because our first and most frequently experienced instinct is located in the stomach, many of the subsequent instinctual feelings which we host are localised in the abdomen. We tend to place our hand on our belly when we are in grief, when we are in shock, when we are consumed with exhilaration and when we are awash with sorrow. And the primary expression of these deep instinctual feelings is vocal; cries, wails, moans, chuckles, guffaws, sobs and yells seem to rise up from the belly and emerge from the mouth.

For the baby, there is a sense of a continuous tube running through the centre of the torso with a hole at both ends: one in the face and one in the buttocks. Prior to conditioning, there is little taboo surrounding what goes in and what comes out of this tube. For the young infant, food is suckled at the lips and passes down the tube into the stomach. But it is just as likely to reemerge back through the mouth as regurgitated liquid as it is likely to be expelled from the anal opening at the other end of the body. Regurgitating food is natural for the baby and is not pathologised by the mother; in fact it often occurs when the baby releases wind from the stomach, often encouraged by the mother's rubbing of the baby's back. However, in time, the infant realises that once food has passed into the body through the mouth and down the tube, it should only exit again at the opposite end. From the point when this has been recognised, a re-emission of food from the mouth is then identified as a sign of pathology: we are only sick when we are ill.

The pre-verbal infant uses the voice to express instinctual feelings and is not yet ready to articulate sounds to communicate thought. However, in time, the instinct to articulate is born and the instinctive sounds of crying, cooing and babbling lead into the formation of the first words which give expression to the formation of the first thoughts. As thought and language develop, the child begins to locate the act of thinking in the head. Indeed, most adults naturally localise the experience of thinking in their head. We touch our brow when in deep thought, but rarely when we are in touch with deep feelings. Whereas instinctual feelings seem to rise up from the belly to emerge from the mouth as sounds, thoughts seem to descend from the head to emerge from the mouth as words. Both feelings and thoughts, then, have to pass through the throat where they feel as though they are converted to sound. This makes the throat a kind of bottleneck, a point of convergence between the two major pathways: the pathway of thoughts which descend from the head and the pathway of feelings which arise from the depths.

The Sonorous Embrace

The mother's voice is the baby's beacon; like a foghorn perched high on the rocky cliffs, it signals the promise of a safe landing upon the shores of an unfamiliar island. In a very short space of time, the mother and baby recognise each other's voice and can easily tell them apart from all other voices. Together they sing a duet which creates a musical enclosure, an orchestral embrace, a sonorous envelope. The baby craves this sonorous envelope because it replaces the lost amniotic haven where the growing babe was supported and surrounded completely. Sound and water behave in similar ways, travelling multidirectionally, filling every chink and every crevice. Like water, sound encloses and enfolds us, surrounding our frame in a complete circle. We can hear a sound emanating from behind us as well as we can hear a sound which originates in front. For a baby craving the lost refuge of the womb, sound offers a gratifying alternative to the amniotic waters. Deaf babies as well as those with healthy auditory canals feel sound across the whole surface of the body. Like Beethoven, who sawed off the legs of his piano and lay upon the ground before it so he could feel the music of his invention quiver and tremor to his bones, babies are astute and alive to the physicality of sound.

When the mother holds the baby in her arms and combines her vocal serenade with the pendulum sway of her body, the sonorous embrace is intensified by the physical hold. But the mother can continue to assure the baby of her presence, even when she is out of contact and out of sight, by continuing to sing and vocalise; for whilst the eyes see a field of vision spanning less than one hundred and eighty degrees, the ears hear an auditory landscape of three hundred and sixty degrees. Through her voice the mother is all around, omnipresent, ubiquitous and enfolding.

When the mother does disappear from the ear, the baby can feel abandoned and isolated and may become highly agitated. But by listening carefully to the mother's voice, the baby learns to copy her inflections and utter little melodies which the young infant sings repeatedly as a way of holding on to the mother's calming presence. Singing becomes an acoustic source of comfort which assuages and conciliates the anxious infant and keeps the mother's voice alive in her temporary absence. Of course, there is a shadow to every light and a discord looming behind every harmony. The relationship between mother and baby is often a din and a pandemonium; and just as the mother's voice can envelop and enfold so it can engulf and enmesh. The ever-present serenade of the mother's tones can become overbearing and eventually all babies will want to silence the source of sound which once they could not do without.

The vocal and physical relationship between mother and child moulds the child's impression of the surrounding environment. Sound makes space; and the quality of sound in a baby's environment, particularly the orchestration of the mother's voice, colours her experience of that space. Some mothers suffer from things which prevent the baby from feeling secure in the company of her voice; and we are all affected by the way in which we were held or not held by our mother's body and our mother's voice. How secure we feel in the arms of the world depends upon how safe we felt in the cradle of the mother's arms and voice.

Cradling is an essential component of the infant's sense of security and containment. Constant and responsive cradling provides a calming, secure and invulnerable arena in which the babe can find amnesty from the harsh impregnations of the hardy world. In cradling, the mother's voice and arms enclose and incubate the baby's body and soul so that the infant can experience the gift of uncompromised support, as though in cradling the mother provides a sensate and palpable experience of unconditional love. But such cradling is an ideal which many mothers cannot be expected to provide and an experience which many infants never receive. Each mother plays host to a pantheon of ghosts and demons, intimidations and misgivings which fill their cradling with a current of unstable and undependable energy which the baby intuits and perceives. And the mother's turmoil is communicated to the baby as much through the acoustic tone of her voice as through the muscle tone of her arms. A sense of insecurity, fear and agitation experienced by the mother can be communicated to the baby through specific vocal timbres, which may give the baby the impression of a container which is unstable, undefined and frail, impeding the baby's own sense of security. A mother's voice which is too penetrative and abrasive may cause the baby to feel intimidated and overwhelmed. A mother's voice which is too timid may leave the baby without a sense of support. Nervousness, irritability, depression and bewilderment can turn the mother's sonata and serenade into a fragmented furore. The mother's entire physiology and psychology is disturbed and highly demanded of by the process of giving birth and nurturing a needy infant; and she is inevitably going to fall short of the ideal mothering that we may invent in the realm of the idea.

My Mother's Tongue

The period of spontaneous vocalising, during which the baby sings out sounds which are innate and inborn, is short lived. For soon the infant must learn to pick and choose. They must terminate the honeymoon of free experimentation and learn to omit some sounds and retain others.

During the early stage of development, the infant combines consonants and vowels musically, emotionally and instinctively, scoring the notes of a universal composition in the air with cries, burps, wheezes, dribbles and cascading tones which erupt from the cradle like a siren. From this experimentation the infant creates a baby-speak, a goo-goo-ga-ga, a jumble-talk, a nonsense language. In other words, the baby creates a concoction of sounds which has no linguistic meaning, yet expresses directly the instincts and emotions of the tiny vocalist.

Though the nonsense language of the infant has no linguistic meaning, it does contain the building blocks for future speech. It is made up of little sound units which the infant must learn to combine into his/her mother's tongue, if s/he is to be accepted as a communicative adult in a world of talk. When listening to a pre-verbal infant combine these units of sound, we are aware of his/her feelings not from what is uttered, which after all is only gobbledegook, but from the musical way in which it is vocalised. Likewise, the infant responds not to the linguistic content of a parent's voice, but to the pitch and tonal colour of the sung tones. The infant's babbling is uttered instinctively, according to a musical or tonal spontaneity in which the entire canvas of the baby's voice, including every vowel, burp and lip-smacking pop are all just various ways of singing to the world. However, the child's success as a potential adult with full communicative faculty depends upon her/his ability to harness this vocal sound-making to a set of laws. The laws which must be obeyed are those which govern the way that spontaneous sounds are combined into words; and the words which must be spoken are those which have meaning in the immediate society which awaits the child just beyond the cradle. Our competence and our intelligence is judged by how well we can say what we mean, even if we do not mean what we say.

The transition from the universal baby-song to the acquisition of the mother tongue specific to the child's culture is achieved by a process of education. The mother, father or person raising the child encourages the sounds which have a place in the words of their language; meanwhile, the caregiver discourages those which their particular language does not utilise, so that the unusable ones become extinct.

The rules of acquired verbal communication change from one context to another, from country to country; and some sounds are accepted in one place or language and not in another. In German, for example, many words end with 'unf', a sound which is not accepted in English. The spoken language of Arabic as well as that of German makes use of the sound 'ach' as in the name of the musical composer Bach; again this sound is not used in English. Yet, all babies from every quarter of the globe make the sounds 'ach' and 'unf' as part of their musical expression.

Through the process of training, the infant's original acoustic tapestry which utilises the entire range of semi-articulate sounds available to a human voice is reduced. Eventually, the only remaining sounds are those which are of linguistic use in the society beyond the cradle. Although on the one hand this process represents progress, it also involves a loss. For the English infant, for example, it means death to the 'unf' and the 'ach'. But there are feelings stored in those sounds. The 'unf' and the 'ach', the gurgles and the cries, the sucking sounds and the blowing sounds all carry pieces of the baby's emerging emotional soul. Now, however, the infant can no longer trust that these feelings will be conveyed through the creative play of sounds which emerge spontaneously from the voice. To secure a response, the child can no longer cry out their emotions, sing out their discomfort, call out their excitement or wail their hunger. Now, the child must translate all such moods and needs into recognisable words.

In the pre-verbal phase, vocal sounds act as a direct expression of experience. With the advent of language, words serve to describe this experience. The word 'sad' replaces the sound of sadness. The word 'joy' replaces the sound of joy. As a result, the actual experience of sadness or joy is no longer necessary to communication. The intensity of such emotions is thereby diluted, as feeling is usurped by thought and vocal sound is replaced with the spoken word. We do not need to feel what we say in order to speak it.

As we enter verbal language we are aware of the price which we pay. Pre-verbal singing seems to express our being and achieve our needs perfectly. But now we must speak clearly for our supper and there seems to be little room for our feelings in the tiny spaces between words. Sound now has no meaning unless it is channelled into speech.

Daddy Holds the Pen

In the traditional triadic setting of mother–father–child, the acquisition of verbal language is complexly interwoven with the significance and increasing presence of the father to the infant.

As the child separates from the mother, it becomes aware of a dialogue and discourse between mother and father which takes place through the medium of verbal language. Furthermore, the child must learn this language if he or she is to enter into the dialogue and, through spoken articulation, secure a place in the family construct which will preserve intimacy with the mother. It is as though the infant gradually recognises that mother and father speak a wholly different language to that spontaneous vocalising which seems to have been exclusive to the intimate mother–infant relationship up until now.

Prior to the acquisition of language, the baby barely notices that they are an entity separate from the mother. But as the acquisition of language and the synonymous separation occur, the infant is able to perceive that he or she is part of an organisation which contains at least two others: mother and father; and possibly siblings also. It is primarily through verbal language that the infant turns from the exclusive pre-verbal semiology of spontaneous vocalisation to the specific codified schema of linguistic signification which it identifies as the medium of discourse which the mother and father use to communicate. In dramatic terms, the infant now enters the scene in which mother and father speak to one another and makes a contribution to this scene through the dexterity of tongue.

Because the baby associates the mother with the pre-verbal plenitude of immediate expression through vocalisation, it naturally, by opposition, associates the father with the law of this new linguistic code. Metaphorically speaking, the father holds the pen: the power to enter the world and penetrate it with the tool of language.

The child is initially dependent upon the mother and father for the rules of this verbal symbology; and these rules always come with the twist of personal psychology, pathology and preference. The way that language acquisition is facilitated in the family is intimately woven into the psychodynamic fabric of the family structure. In particular, because of the association of linguistic power and the paternal law, the father's own dictates and legislations play a particularly influential part in shaping the emotional and psychological atmosphere surrounding the use of verbal language. But both the mother and father together create a set of psychological rules which intersect with the linguistic rules and which are passed on to the child as the language of adult discourse.

Every family is structured around a set of rules, a legislation which dictates what is permissible and what is forbidden; and this includes taboos regarding what can and cannot be spoken. The infant, who is at first innocent of these laws, has to learn the code of the family; and part of this learning involves the shocking recognition that not all that the child thinks and feels inside is welcome. Of course, each family has its own taboos: some will not tolerate blasphemy; some will not accept talking about sex; others will not allow members of the family to voice their opinion about other members; some parents will not permit the child to argue a point of contention or disagreement; other families frown upon the expression of emotion. In other families, the laws are more insidious or confusing and what can be voiced to one parent must be kept a secret from the other.

Prior to the acquisition of verbal language, there is little restraining the infant from an immediate expression of feeling, sensation and desire. Now, however, these must be harnessed to a sophisticated psychological acoustic code which combines the original emotionality of voice with the new cognition of words.

Sub-text and Undertones

Oral communication between adults is composed of two dimensions: voice and speech. The term 'voice' refers to the sound produced by the vibrating vocal cords. The term 'speech' refers to the shaping of these sounds into words by articulating the mouth, lips, jaw and tongue. In fact, the term 'linguistic' comes from *lingua*, the Latin word for tongue. The sound of the voice, independent of the words uttered, is composed of different ingredients such as pitch, loudness, register, free air and nasality, which combine in different proportions to form a range of tonal colours or timbres; and the tonal colour of the voice acts as the messenger for our state of mind, moods, emotions and inner attitudes. Most people are quite aware that the same spoken phrase can be uttered in such a variety of voices as to communicate significantly different meanings. In the words of a common but wise adage: 'It is not what you say but the way that you say it'.

The voice dimension to oral communication reveals much about the personality of the speaker and a change in tonal colour can completely alter the meaning of the same verbal sentence, imbuing it with passivity or ferocity, ecstasy or despair. In the timbral quality of a voice you can hear the vales of depression and the peaks of excitement, you can hear the lulls of concern and self-reflection and the sharp points of provocation and attack; in it you can hear the calm tone of age and wisdom and the effervescent innocence and enthusiasm of youth; in the voice you can hear resignation, indignation, hope and despair. In short, in the voice you can hear the psyche.

Although the voice may give speech its emotional meaning, it does not necessarily simply enforce the verbal content. For example, if the speaker is in some kind of personal conflict, the two channels may carry contradictory information. This is called incongruence and often occurs when the words we choose paint a public face which disguises our true feelings. We say that we are willing to do something for a friend with a tone of voice which reveals a reluctance to help; we say that we are feeling fine whilst we are actually choked with sadness. When such an incongruence between the vocal and verbal message occurs, the voice is more likely to reveal the truth about the personality than the speech.

A common kind of incongruence can often be heard in the acoustic messages conveyed to children by their parents.

Case Study: Michael

Leaving Mother

Michael was an only child who was raised by a single mother. The mother was frail, lonely and dependent upon her son for company. Whenever the son announced that he was going out alone, to spend time with a friend or to take part in the social activities befitting his age, his mother's words would wish him well and encourage him on his way. However, her tone of voice would give Michael the impression that she really didn't want him to go. This had made it very difficult for Michael to leave his mother; even as an adult, he felt that in some way he ought to be at home looking after her. Michael found it very difficult to be clear about his needs, particularly in his relationships with women. He would want affection but convey an attitude of cold detachment;

he would wish to bring a relationship to an end, but continue to humour someone, too afraid to be clear about his feelings.

There are many amongst us who have been raised on a staple diet of confused and ambivalent messages. As a result, we in turn can find it hard to convey a single intention or feeling. Instead, we paint one picture with the words we speak and another with our vocal intonation.

Case Study: Teri
A Sweet Voice for Daddy

Just as a child's needs are directed towards the mother, so too every mother has needs which she hopes her child will fulfil. Every mother wants something from the baby she nurtures. And the same may be said for fathers.

Teri, whose case I explored in the previous chapter, came to work on herself through Voice Movement Therapy because she felt her voice was too high in pitch, too breathy and too childlike. She hoped that the work might enable her to lower the pitch of her voice and enable her to sound 'more mature'. At the same time, she was a little worried because her boyfriend liked her voice and she was concerned that she might lose his affections if her voice changed too much.

As Teri explained her story I noticed that her speaking voice did create the impression of naivete and susceptibility; and her entire demeanour was very pubescent. This was compounded by her short summer frock, her pink shoes and her long blond hair which hung in pigtails tied with ribbons.

It seemed to me that, in order to retain the father's love, Teri had maintained a voice which was quiet, high in pitch, in flute timbre and falsetto register, and which she felt created the acoustic image of the sweet little girl that her father demanded in return for his love. Teri remained a little girl for her father and from here she went into a relationship with an older man who encouraged her to express herself through the same childlike sweetness as her father had done.

A Voice to Please Another Ear

We are all susceptible to the demands which others make of us; and these demands can often become manifest in the way that we give voice in the world. Many infants have had to guess what the mother and father seek in the child and then produce the desired expression in order to obtain the rewards of comfort, food and nurturing. Often, this 'second guessing' carries on into adult life where many people subconsciously express that which they believe the other party expects or desires. In acoustic terms, this is equivalent to voicing that which we believe the other wishes to hear rather than that which we believe expresses the authenticity of our inner thoughts and feelings. For those who are entrenched in this pattern, their true voice often becomes lost, buried and forgotten and their psyche becomes orientated around echoing the others with whom they relate. For those such as Teri, where such a pattern is scored deep into the early childhood history, uncovering the voices of the true selves can be exhilarating and shocking.

The process of echoing that which we perceive to be desired is one of two major psychophonic complexes found amongst adults in therapy. The second is a condition which we may call phonophobia.

Phonophobia

Phonophobia is literally a fear of voicing and the phonophobic child, though capable of speaking up and speaking out, does so under great duress, terrified that they may say the wrong thing. Beneath this phobia is often a worry that in speaking out they will betray the code of the family and make private knowledge public news. Often, children carry this phonophobic condition through into adulthood when they appear as shy, reticent and uncertain of their words. But although phonophobic people seem quiet on the outside, their inner world is often an orchestra of sound. During conversation, their thoughts and feelings swirl round and round in their head like a barrel organ. They know what they think and what they feel; they have an opinion and an elaborate perspective. But between the mind and the throat there is an iron door through which nothing can escape. The phonophobic smiles sweetly and says a simple and agreeable 'ah ah'.

Those Who are Made Mute

To understand the phonophobic's voice which is soft and easily drowned by the cacophony of the crowd, it is useful to examine the extreme example of phonophobia or voicelessness: mutism. Mutism comes from the Latin *mutos* meaning silent and the person suffering from mutism is literally struck dumb. Total mutism is quite rare, but when it does occur its roots are nearly always psychological. The vocal cords can vibrate, the mouth can articulate and the mind is awash with complex thoughts and deep feelings. But between the conception and the sound, between the emotion and the word falls a shadow of silence: the mute is dumb-struck. Though total mutism is quite rare, elective mutism is relatively common and is a condition of intermittent silence where a child is perfectly fluent of speech in some circumstances yet seemingly dumb in others. Some children may go mute at school but speak clearly at home. Other children may go mute only when in the presence of doctors and nurses or when left alone with a stranger or when in a large group.

Speech therapists and psychologists working with electively mute children have discovered that many of these young people are guarding a secret which they are afraid of betraying. Rather than risk the hidden knowledge slipping out amidst a trail of harmless words, they close down altogether until they are back in the safe company of those with whom they share the secret.

Case Study: Jane
Silent Secrets

Jane was a classic example of a child who kept quiet to avoid spilling the beans. She lived in a large household with her four older sisters and brothers, her parents and her grandparents. Shortly after Jane's birth her mother suffered post-natal depression which developed into a mental illness characterised by irrational and bizarre behaviour, radical changes of mood and vitriolic verbal abuse directed at the grandparents.

When Jane was old enough to ask her grandmother what was wrong with her mummy, she was told: 'Mummy got sick trying to push you out of her tummy and used herself all up trying to look after you.' Understandably, Jane blamed herself for her mother's illness and when a therapist asked her if she felt it was her fault that her mother became mentally ill, Jane replied: 'Well, of course, if I hadn't come along she would be alright.'

When Jane was old enough to begin playing with other children at their homes, her father instructed her to 'never utter a word' about her mother's illness. When Jane began school, these instructions were repeated with greater vehemence when her grandmother told her: 'When you are at school you make sure you say nothing about your mother.' For a young child this amounts to saying nothing at all. For, what child can talk without referring to the most significant person in their life? In Jane's case, she did the only thing that could guarantee her ability to satisfy her grandmother's instructions. She said nothing at all when at school. Not a word. With her friends on her street she spoke, but with decreasing fluency until her speech degenerated into single word answers. Eventually, she spoke only between the walls of her own house.

Mental illness in the family creates an awful stigma and causes a lot of shame; and the relatives of the sick person can spend as much energy disguising and camouflaging it as they can seeking to heal it. Mental illness also attracts a spectrum of descriptions from the inane to the horrific. The person suffering a mental illness is having a 'nervous breakdown'; they are 'cracking up' or 'falling apart'; they have a 'screw loose', have 'lost their marbles' and gone 'over the edge'. They are mad, insane and demented. These abominable words make it very difficult for a family to discuss the psychological troubles of a loved one and can leave parents bereft of knowing what to say to the children. The so-called professional language of psychiatric diagnoses is no better and has barely changed since the days of asylums and straight-jackets. Labels like 'senile dementia', 'schizophrenia' and 'manic depression' are blanket terms used to cover such a wide spectrum of individual problems that two people with the same diagnoses may have absolutely nothing in common. It is hard to speak of mental suffering when we lack a compassionate vocabulary for psychological problems. Because of the stigma surrounding mental illness, which is made worse by the language many people use to describe it, the priority of many families is to keep the news from spreading. For the children, this means staying loyal to a code of secrets and lies and avoiding any reference to the psychological difficulties within the family when in public.

The Unspeakable Subject of Dying

Another subject which a family can find difficult to speak of is death. Death is a skeleton in everyone's cupboard. It lurks with inevitable certainty and yet we talk little of it as though somehow, by leaving it unspoken, we can stave off its coming. When we do speak of death it is often dressed in fear, insecurity and unease. And when our children ask us to give death a name and a face, a rhyme and a reason, we are often quite literally lost for words. The way we present death to children shapes their understanding of what it means to live. If children are offered an explanation which is both truthful yet hopeful, they can grow to accept the only sure event which each of us is guaranteed to encounter. But if we describe death as a finality without a future or if we pretend it does not in some way represent an end, the child can only be troubled, confused and bewildered.

One of the reasons that death can be so difficult to explain is that it is a subject which calls us to expose and declare our fundamental spiritual beliefs. For the family with a strong religious foundation, this is hard enough. But for parents whose spiritual life is underdeveloped or unconsidered, knowing what to say to a grief-ridden child when a family member dies is a serious problem. In extreme cases, parents do manage to avoid admitting to the child that a death has occurred and instead they pretend that the deceased family member has temporarily taken a journey and will eventually return.

Case Study: Julian

Your Brother's Gone Away

When one of my clients called Julian was five years old, his older brother died in a road accident. Julian did not see the body and did not attend the funeral. When he asked his parents where his brother was, they told him that he had gone away to a special school because he was so clever. Julian repeatedly asked when they could visit his brother but was answered with false promises and excuses. Like Jane, Julian was told 'not to breathe a word' about his brother at school, because the other children would be jealous. Like Jane, Julian became mute for a considerable period. He would not talk to teachers, to friends or to doctors. He would talk only to relatives.

The Loyalty of Youth

Both Jane and Julian were silenced by their loyalty. Rather than risk breaking the family code of privacy, they stopped speaking altogether.

Loyalty is probably the child's most developed instinct; it easily matches the maternal instinct of protection. Even children who are abused by one of their parents will display a loyalty to the family as though by instinct. No matter how harsh, how confusing, how unfair and how destructive, the family is the child's first and last bastion. Children will wage war against the world at large with lies, with protest, with cleverly constructed cover-up stories and, if necessary, with complete and utter silence, rather than betray the hand that feeds – even if that hand also threatens.

Julian and Jane are extreme cases and not all children who guard a family secret become electively mute. But many children become caught in a web of conflict and confusion about what they should and should not say and suffer a milder form of voicelessness in the form of phonophobia.

When John and Jane came to work through Voice Movement Therapy they were in their early forties and the mutism of their childhood was far behind them. But, they both came seeking help because they felt terribly blocked in their ability to speak out; and it is such difficulties for which Voice Movement Therapy is ideally suited. And one of the reasons that Voice Movement Therapy can be instrumental in dismantling phonophobia and other psychogenic vocal inhibitions is that it provides a structure within which the original conditions and circumstances which instigated the phonophobia can be revisited.

Practical Method: Recalling the Family Voices

Clients are asked to reflect upon the nature of their parents' voices and the voices of any siblings, and to consider how they sounded. It is useful to ask clients to recline on the floor with their eyes closed and to try and conjure an acoustic memory of their mother's and father's voice and the voices of brothers and sisters from their childhood days.

Focusing particularly on the parents, clients are asked to recall specific turns of phrases and vocal mannerisms which typify the parents' vocal habits. As the client muses, it is useful for them to try and recall how their parents responded vocally to specific situations: when the client was ill, when the client was angry or bored, when the client was defiant or joyous. Usually, clients are able to remember very specific verbal and vocal details which have become scored into the client's psyche like a song.

Clients are then asked to notate the acoustic ingredients of their parents' voices using the Voice Movement Therapy system. If clients remember a parent using a particular combination of ingredients under certain circumstances that were different to the usual colour of the voice, then they are asked to notate these also.

Case Study: Martin

No Room to Voice

Martin, whom I first introduced in Volume One of this series (Newham 1999a), was thirty-six; he was married with two children and had driven a taxi for twelve years. His reason for attending Voice Movement Therapy was that he had what he described as a 'stutter' which no previous endeavour had succeeded in alleviating. He found it difficult to remember exactly when he developed a 'stutter', but he felt that it was around the age of eight. I noticed at first that his 'stutter' was irregular and vowels were as equally affected as consonants. However, the most striking thing about Martin's speech pattern was the involuntary jerking movements of his head and neck which accompanied vocalisation and which were particularly exaggerated during his 'stuttering'. His eyes closed, the head tilted backwards and to one side, the neck stiffened and his facial muscles contorted. His head would then jerk rhythmically and spasmodically for the duration of the interrupted sound. The look upon his face during such episodes was, to my personal eyes, one of tremendous fear. Then, on further listening to the so-called 'stuttered' sounds, I noticed that in fact what was happening was more adequately described as a kind of contorted gagging of the larynx. The sounds which occurred during this balking were in flute timbre and sounded strained and contracted; and he described that it felt as though 'air could not get out'. I therefore became convinced that the majority of Martin's speech difficulties originated not in what would be clinically described as a 'stammer', which causes a 'trip over words', but in a constriction of the pharynx and larynx. The amount of times he stumbled over consonants made with tongue or lips were actually very few, but the gagging occurred with all vowels as well as with certain consonants, particularly 'k', during which he would extend the sound into a gurgling noise which, if I refrained from witnessing the fearful expression on Martin's face, reminded me of a baby regurgitating or expelling unwanted milk.

Martin could not locate any single incident in his life which he could describe as severely traumatic. However, he spoke about his relationship to his father as having been a source of ongoing trauma. His father was a devout and extremely strict Catholic and a professor of chemistry; his other two sons were both doctors. It had been clear from quite an early age that Martin was not going to reveal the same predisposition to academic activity as the rest of his family. Another significant memory for Martin, was that he had been the brunt of jokes made by his peers at school and by his brothers at home, who called him 'bunny' because he had an involuntary twitch in his cheek. And, though Martin could not locate any single traumatic event, it became obvious over the period of our work together that his entire childhood had been a very unhappy one. Not only did he grow up in the shadow of his brothers' achievements, but he also had a mother who showed him little attention and no physical affection. He could not remember ever being held or cuddled or kissed by his mother; furthermore, he never saw his parents hold hands or show any physical signs of love to one another. The picture of his family life that emerged was an incredibly sterile one. Dry academic conversations, competitive brothers, meals at regular times often with guests who would parade their expert intellectual preoccupations, and a mother with a cool and distant relationship to her sons and her husband.

When I first met Martin I had asked if he had any other illnesses or difficulties apart from what he described as his 'stutter'. Martin had replied that he had for many years suffered periodically from extreme headaches. He dealt with them by taking a variety of analgesics but they rarely alleviated what he described as the 'sensation of pressure between his temples'. On investigating further the genesis of these headaches it was revealed that they worsened during times of extended verbal activity; the more he 'stuttered' the more his head ached.

Martin liked his job as a taxi driver because 'on a bad day' he could 'get away' without talking to anyone. However, on a good day he would enjoy chatting to his customers and was frustrated intensely because he felt the 'stutter' was preventing him from partaking of the social activities which he enjoyed. Martin was also keen to point out that as a taxi driver he frequently escorted customers of some importance – 'scientists', 'writers', 'actors' and others whom he described as having 'made it'. When asked to describe how he thought such people perceived him when he 'stuttered', Martin was categorical that he appeared 'stupid'. The words he used to describe the way he thought that he was perceived included 'daft', 'idiotic', 'a moron' and a 'dim-wit'. It emerged that these were all words which his brothers had used against him.

It also emerged gradually that Martin had associated verbal proficiency with intelligence. The fact that he had not 'lived up' to the academic standing of his father and brothers had made him feel stupid and his voice problem further compounded this feeling and in many ways became a symbol for it. It was also clear that Martin wanted sympathy for his condition, and indeed he responded very eagerly to a sympathetic attitude. In this respect he had very clear memories of his grandmother. She had been a very important figure in his life as a child and a single source of comfort, understanding and physical affection; she had also been very kind about his 'stutter'. It was also his grandmother who had told him that when he was born the doctors had told his mother that he was 'much too small and light' and that she should rectify this by feeding him twelve bottles of milk per day. Martin had therefore been awakened from sleep continually as an infant and had been force-fed with milk.

The first stage of Martin's journey, which I have outlined in Volume One of this series (Newham 1999a), involved using the physical and respiratory aspects of Voice Movement Therapy to overcome the stammering and release a fluent voice, which he achieved successfully. He also overcame the persistent headaches.

However, once the stammer had subsided, though Martin was left with a fluent voice, he experienced incredible reticence about giving voice in public and began to suffer from a persistent phonophobia. It was clear to Martin that the foundations of his voice problem were rooted in his childhood environment. For Martin, therefore, the process of exploring the family voices offered him a welcomed opportunity to recover from an age-old pattern of vocal inhibition.

Client's Account: Martin

A Day at the Opera

I found the exercise of recalling the family voices very stirring. When I checked the clock after lying on the floor for what seemed like only five minutes, I realised I had been doing the exercise for nearly half an hour. It was like revisiting the family world of my childhood. I could remember meal times specifically and the sound of my mother's and father's voice – so measured, so controlled, so sweet to one another, yet underneath a certain cold acerbic frustration.

I had no trouble recording the vocal ingredients. My father's voice was loud, low pitch, modal register, saxophone timbre with attack. My mother's voice was quiet, high pitch, modal register, flute timbre with free air. Had they been singers they would have produced marvellous duets.

Whilst lying on the floor with my eyes closed, the overwhelming feeling was of being an audience to their relationship, like at the theatre or the opera, with no way of entering into the dialogue. Yet, I also had clear visions of them parting the waves and both asking me what I thought about something and me just sitting there not knowing what to say. The word that came to mind was intimidation. As I realised this, I became quite tearful at the thought of being so excluded and so intimidated by my own parents. And when I came to sit up and do the notation, my eyes were wet. I could not help wondering what I did with all my tears when I was little. I think I buried them.

Case Study: Janice

Rape and Silence

Janice, whom I also first introduced in Volume One of this series (Newham 1999a), was a professional musician whose primary instrument was and is the French horn.

At the height of her career when she was enjoying success as a much sought after player, Janice was consecutively raped by three men one night on her way home after a concert. Two of the three men took turns to hold her to the ground whilst the other raped her.

Despite the severe physical pain and the extreme emotional shock, Janice could barely make a sound throughout her ordeal. She tried to scream but could only produce a muffled shout. Whenever her voice did get anywhere near being loud enough to be heard, her oppressors covered her mouth with their hands.

As a result of her ordeal, Janice was unable to play with the orchestra for ten months, during which time she received counselling twice a week.

Since the ordeal she had suffered three main physical symptoms: a feeling that she had an iron bar running vertically down the centre of her torso, a feeling of constriction around the throat and constant breathlessness. In addition, her voice felt paralysed.

The first stage of Janice's work, which I have outlined in Volume One of this series (Newham 1999a), involved using the physical and respiratory aspects of Voice Movement Therapy to overcome the feeling of vocal paralysis, release the constriction around the larynx and alleviate the feeling of rigidity down the chest. For Janice, this was accompanied by some major cathartic experiences during which extreme sounds in the form of groans, screams and shrieks were released in combination with aggressive and wild bodily movements.

The second stage of Janice's work, which I have outlined in *Using Voice and Song in Therapy* (Newham 1999b), involved transforming the vocal sounds which arose from her catharsis into consciously composed songs which provided a container and an opportunity for healing through creativity.

As a result of these two stages, Janice felt that she had overcome the major inhibitions arising as a result of her tragic ordeal. In this final stage of her work, Janice wanted to revisit her family life to see if she could discover why she had experienced a reaction to being raped that involved introverted withdrawal and silence, rather than extroverted anger and intensified expressivity. For she felt that somehow her mother and father had not encouraged the females in the family to express themselves vocally, particularly where anger or aggression was concerned.

Client's Account: Janice

Voice for the Boys, Music for the Girls

I lay on the floor for about forty minutes recapturing the acoustic environment of my early years. The picture was of me and my sister practising our musical instruments for the next exam whilst my two brothers had deep and meaningful conversations with my father.

I remember my father's voice very clearly. It was a light high voice: quiet, high pitch, clarinet timbre with free air. An unusual voice for a man but very distinctive and distinguished.

Though I remember my father's voice very clearly, I cannot remember ever talking to him very much. This seemed to be reserved for the boys. Sometimes, my two brothers and my father would get quite heated – especially around anything political. They were, in fact, encouraged to express their opinions and my father seemed to relish the argumentative spirit in them. But my sister and I were always expected to be 'lady like' and were often scolded for 'raising our voices'. In fact, one of my father's often used lines towards me was: 'If you have energy to shout young lady you have energy to practise your horn'. It seems so ridiculous now, but I accepted it then.

My mother's voice was louder and deeper than my father's. Her voice was loud, middle pitch, modal register, flute timbre with a moderate amount of violin and attack. Unlike my father, she did not enjoy any kind of energetic discourse and would ask 'the men' to keep their voices down when a heated debate was taking place. I can never remember my mother showing any emotion. When anything tragic happened, she responded with protracted silence. I remember when her mother died she hardly said a word for about three weeks and then bounced back as though the curtains had been drawn and the light was beaming through the window once again.

As I lay on the floor touring my family, I recalled event after event where I had my voice tempered: times when I would rush in after school with some exciting news only to be told to calm down before speaking. Times when I was deeply upset about something and told to dry my eyes and accept it as 'part of life's rich tapestry'. I can remember being told this long before I knew what a 'tapestry' was. And, I could also remember times when I was furious about something – particularly during my young adolescence when I became quite political and environmentally conscious. My mother's response was always to tell me to 'hush' and accept it. My father's response was always to tell me to play out my fury upstairs in the music room where I might improve my playing at the same time.

When I came to sit up and notate the ingredients of my parents' and brothers' and sister's voices, it began to dawn on me that my reaction to the rape was the reaction I had been programmed to have: quiet withdrawal and acceptance. Only this time, I could not go up to the music room and play it away – I was far too hurt. I simply could not play my horn. It was almost as though there was a kind of defiance in this too. As though this time I was going to refuse to simply express myself through my instrument – I needed to voice my pain. Only then could I return to my horn out of my own choice, rather than because no other voice was afforded me.

Practical Method: Recording the Parental Voices

This exercise is only possible where the parents of the client are still alive.

The client is asked to think about a subject which would form an appropriate topic of conversation to explore with their parents. It is useful to choose something which would be of genuine interest to the parents and about which they are likely to have opinions.

Clients are asked to make a visit to their parents and to explain to them that they are pursuing a project which involves studying the human voice. The client then asks the parents for permission to make a tape recording of their voices and sets up a microphone and recording machine ready to begin. The client then interviews the parents, acting as both chairperson and contributor, encouraging the parents to speak freely so that the fabric and timbre of their voices are given a chance to be expressed.

For the next stage of the investigation, the client takes some private solo time to listen to the recording made of the parents' voices and reflects upon how the voices have changed and how they have remained the same. In particular, clients are asked to reflect upon how it felt to be in a triadic conversation with the parents now, compared to how they recalled the feeling of communicating with the parents as a child when laying on the floor in the earlier exercise.

Practical Method: The Radio Play

In this next stage of the exploration, each client is asked to create a radio play with the following three characters: the client as a child, the client's mother and the client's father.

Clients are asked to recall the quality of dialogue which existed between their parents, drawing on memories of times when the family were together, such as meal times around the table or a journey in a car. The client also draws upon the audio recording which has been made.

The client is asked to try and recall the specific quality of the parents' voices, their vocal mannerisms and turns of phrases, the way they answered each other. The client tries to recapture the feeling of being a child and to get some recollection of how their voice contributed to the ambience and structure of inter-family communication.

The client then writes the script for a five-minute radio play which epitomises and encapsulates the essence of the vocal dialogue between the three characters as remembered by the client.

The client then rehearses the radio play giving each of the three characters a specific vocal quality by combining ingredients of the Voice Movement Therapy system.

On returning to the group, each member then performs the radio play, playing each of the three characters and executing appropriate sound effects, witnessed by the group.

Client's Account: Janice

Performing the radio play was like putting the pieces of a jigsaw together and finally seeing a clear picture. Though I had come into therapy with the hope of overcoming the symptoms I had suffered since I had been raped, this work took me deeper and gave me insight into why I had developed those particular symptoms.

When I played the part of my mother, I felt so much like her and found myself coughing in the way she used to cough all the time. She also used to tap her chest simultaneously. I wondered if the feeling I had in my chest after being raped and the tightness in my throat was somehow an extreme version of what she felt all the time. When I played her part for the radio play I had this incredible feeling of there being so much more to be expressed, but of it all being pushed down, as though she needed to get something off her chest but never gave herself permission. It made me realise that the cathartic release I had experienced through therapy was not just a release of the pain experienced as a result of being raped, but of a whole backlog of emotions which I had never been allowed to voice in the family. Giving voice to my mother for the radio play led me to believe that she too had a well of unvoiced emotion in her.

When I played my father's part, I felt so powerful and manipulative, as though I could control the whole family with just a few words. It was as though assuming his voice was like an excuse to execute all the powers which he himself had denied me through his own dogma. I found my voice to be extremely powerful and heard myself use sounds and inflections which I had hitherto never used.

Whereas when I played my mother, I felt like her. With my father, I felt a million miles from being like him. This was reflected in my voice. I found it hard to manifest the combination of vocal ingredients which I had allotted to him, whereas the quality of my mother's voice was easy to reproduce. However, once I found my father's voice it was like a new lease of life, as though I had found a part of my voice which was too shy to come out when he was around.

The overall experience of performing the radio play left me with an incredible feeling of energy. A mixture of anger and determination. I realised that the way that my mother and father had encouraged me to deal with emotions was not going to work for me any more and that – as much as I love playing music – I could no longer use my horn as a substitute for what I needed to voice from my own gut, my own chest and through my own vocal cords.

From Radio to Musical Theatre

The radio play is one of many performance genres which have an emphasis on vocal expression and which can be used in group therapy to facilitate a personal exploration of the psyche within a creative structure.

The radio play is, of course, particularly focused on an investigation of the original family environment within which the voice of the client is shaped. But there are other genres which open up avenues of exploration which the client can use to focus on particular issues specific to their own therapeutic enquiry. One of the main genres which Voice Movement Therapy utilises is Musical Theatre and it is to this genre and its application in Voice Movement Therapy that I will now turn my attention in the following chapter.

CHAPTER 6

The Therapy of Musical Theatre
Using Vocal Performance to Transform the Self

Voice, Theatre and Transformation

The voice provides a medium through which transformation can occur. The voice is, essentially, a transformative instrument. The voice is an acoustic mirror which, unlike the flat and unpliable surface of an optical mirror, is malleable and supple and can refract, compress and rarefy the sound waves which it reflects to create a wholly new sound. And this new sound contains within it the structural basis for the development of new parts of the Self.

The art of transformation is central to both therapy and theatre. In therapy, the client enters a hall of acoustic mirrors which echo and reflect back the voices of the many selves, enabling the client to move expressively between different potentialities. In theatre, the actor delves deep into their soul and allows their expressive instrument to transform into another character.

In ancient Greece, the great theatre festivals were mounted in honour of the god Dionysus who represented the power of transformation. These festivals would coincide with the opening of the new season's wine, formed miraculously from the transformation of grapes. Meanwhile, upon the stage, actors donned masks and, in so doing, would magically transform into heroes, heroines, gods and goddesses. And in the auditorium, the witnesses to this spectacle would experience an emotional transformation through catharsis.

Theatre is an arena of transformation where subject matter is given a fresh voice; and in theatre forms where the expressiveness of the human voice plays a major role – such as opera and musical theatre – subject matter is often radically transformed from one perspective to another.

For example, in the Western world opera has long been regarded as both the most elite and the most exquisite example of high art in which all that is beautiful of form is brought together to make a spectacle of light, colour, costume, music and, above all, vocal dexterity. The opera is perhaps the last bastion of refuge for the concept of aesthetic beauty. Yet, the subject matter of opera is usually almost the opposite to that which society finds beautiful: rape, murder, lust, greed, suicide, oppression, theft and lies. There is in the vast majority of opera a fundamental paradox or contention between the beauty of its form and the ugliness of its content. Opera dresses foul deed in fair form and parades it before an audience who applaud the musical composition and the vocal splendour. Yet, often the story which is being applauded is one involving the suffering of one human being at the hands of another.

To a lesser extent, the same may be said of many musical theatre shows, such as *Sweeney Todd*. Here, again, beautifully costumed performers sing songs with infectious melodies and with grand voices which entertain an audience and move them to laughter and tears. Yet the story told is that which, outside the theatre, one might not consider appropriate to find entertaining.

The use of voice in this theatre of aesthetic paradox is philosophically crucial. For the literal voice of the performer gives a fresh psychological voice to a subject matter. Theatre turns things upside down and leaves no subject beyond its grasp. In therapy this aesthetic paradox is extremely useful. For it provides the client with a precedent for taking their material and using it as the basis of performance which in itself provides a transformative experience. In other words, when personal tragedy is turned into art, into song and lyrics, the illusion of an ultimate exorcism of pain is replaced with the less naive but equally healing practice of artistic transformation. This mechanism sits at the historical heart of artistic process; many artists have composed and painted, written and performed as a way of making something expressive and positive from something inwardly burdensome. Many great artists, and vocalists particularly, have endured life-long sufferings: they have been abused, beaten, degraded; they have lost loved ones in terrible accidents; they have fallen ill to eating disorders and disease; they have been imprisoned and enslaved. The truly great vocalist continues to sing in moments of the greatest and most personalised emotion. The vocalist makes their tragedies public by elevating them to the level of universal relevance. The voice takes a personal event and an idiosyncratic image and turns it into an archetypal form. The vocalist suffers but their voice does not suffer as a result. Suffering may not be necessary in order to give voice; but suffering is no reason not to vocalise – it is the best reason.

We cannot rewrite our history. The traumas which we have befallen in the past are etched upon our souls and no healing can rewrite history. But the voice tricks history by succumbing to its immovable presence. Vocalising writes and rewrites the past. The song remains the same; it can be sung a million times by a million people. To give voice to that which has disempowered us means that at some level we have overcome it.

But finding the tune or melody for a song is only the tip of the iceberg vocally and therapeutically. For, the main therapeutic value in the use of the singing voice rests in the particular quality, colour or timbre of voice with which the tune is sung.

The second healing factor which theatre provides is that it transforms the idiosyncratic experience of a single person into the product of community collaboration and co-operation. To make theatre is to communicate, first to one's fellow performers and second to an audience. The tragedy is no longer resident in the house of the individual psyche. In order for theatre to communicate, the subject matter which may have originated in the psyche of a single individual must have sufficient in common with the psyches of others in order for the spectacle of presentation to weave its healing spell.

Practical Method: Creating and Performing an Opera

First, clients are introduced to the vocal map of Western classical singing. The best way of doing this is to play to the group some excerpts from different operas and break the voices down into the Voice Movement Therapy system of ingredients described in Chapter Three.

The most dominant ingredients in classical opera are very fast pitch fluctuation – or vibrato – with falsetto register dominant in the female voice and modal register in the male voice.

Clients are then asked to experiment with manufacturing these ingredients and producing their impersonation of an 'operatic voice'. This is usually a great deal of fun and clients are often amazed that, through impersonation alone, they can produce a sound which compares to that which they heard in the excerpts.

In the next stage, clients are introduced to different forms of vocal expression within opera, primarily, the solo aria and the duet.

Then, clients are asked to take an event from their life, usually something that they have been working on during the therapeutic process, and to write an opera in three acts for approximately four people. Clients are not required to compose using written musical notation, but simply to write the words and to experiment with melody using the practical method called prosody to melody that I have outlined in Volume Two of this series (Newham 1999b). This method is founded on the simple fact that speech is articulated with a certain prosody. Prosody is the music which underpins language, it is the rise and fall in pitch which brings attitude and implication to what we say and engages the listener in a way that monotone would not. Melody is merely exaggerated prosody, and because everybody uses prosody quite naturally, everyone has the potential ability to create melodies and make songs from their creative writing.

The method used for finding a melody for creative writing in Voice Movement Therapy consists of gradually exaggerating the prosody of the spoken voice into a melody.

It is important that clients are given time to do this, usually three weeks between therapeutic sessions. Then, on returning with their written opera, clients form into groups of about four people and allot a period of time to rehearse and produce each member's opera. Usually, rehearsals continue over a period of some weeks. In each rehearsal and production process, the client responsible for writing the opera at hand acts as director and leads the other members towards executing the opera in a way which satisfies the client.

At the end of the production process, each opera is performed for the witnessing therapeutic group.

Song and Speech in Musical Theatre

Unlike the opera, musical theatre combines both spoken and sung voice. And, this, combined with incongruence and paradox of form and content, adds to its mystery. For, in one moment two people may be involved in a spoken conversation somewhat resembling that which we may hear on the street; and in the next moment the speakers burst into song. Yet the audience receive this blatant transformation from one medium to the other as nothing but expected and ordinary.

In therapy this is again very useful, for to speak of something and to sing of something are not the same – both bring a different voice to the same subject. To provide clients with the opportunity to employ both the speaking and the singing voice to express a subject therefore opens the doors to two different perspectives on the same theme.

Practical Method: Creating a Piece of Musical Theatre

This process is similar to the previous practical method except that the form being investigated is musical theatre. To begin, clients are played excerpts from popular musicals. They are also encouraged to go and see some complete musicals in their own time. In playing the examples to clients, it is useful to point out the use of the relationship between spoken and singing voice. Clients are asked to contemplate what happens to their experience of the subject matter as it passes from spoken to sung text.

Clients are then asked to take an event or a series of situations from their life – usually ones which they have been working on during the therapeutic process – and to write a piece of musical theatre in three scenes for approximately four players. Again, clients are permitted to write their piece in whichever form they choose and to trust the process of rehearsal to bring the piece alive.

Practical Method: Rehearsing a Piece of Musical Theatre

When the pieces have been written, clients form groups of about four people and allot time to rehearsing each member's musical. The person responsible for writing the musical acts as director and brings the piece to fruition. During the rehearsal, the director is asked to utilise the Voice Movement Therapy system to experiment with giving different characters specific vocal qualities. They are also asked to help the performers make transitions between one set of vocal ingredients and another to support the emotional and figurative expressions. This also encourages the client and other performers to experience three different perspectives on the same material. There are a thousand ways of singing the same melody for there are a thousand different qualities of voice with which a tune can be sung. And it is to a large extent the colour or quality or timbre of a voice which carries its emotional content. Therefore, once a client has discovered the means with which to create a melody from prosody, the next and most crucial step is to enable them to access a broad range of vocal qualities which in turn enable the sung and spoken text to be imbued with a diversity of emotion.

Then, the client is asked to prepare three alternative presentations of the same piece, each one using different vocal ingredients. This means that the performers present the piece three times, but in each presentation they will sing the songs and articulate the dialogue with completely different vocal qualities. This naturally influences the emotional tone of the performance.

The group is also asked to collaborate in finding and creating costume props for the production, which may also change from rendition to rendition to bring a different perspective to the same piece.

At the end of the production process, the pieces are performed for the witness therapeutic group. After the three performances of each piece, the witnessing group is asked to comment on the different emotional experience which they received in response to the three pieces. This reveals the way that specific vocal colourings of phrases, words and melodies contribute to the communication of different affects.

The Culmination of Therapeutic Process: Vicky

It is appropriate that the description of the Musical Theatre method comes in the final chapter of the last in a series of three books on the application of Voice Movement Therapy. For the process of creating a theatrical presentation using the Voice Movement Therapy principles is a task which is most suitable as a culmination of a therapeutic process, where material has been worked in many different ways and on many different levels.

In order to show how the Musical Theatre presentation can act as a culmination to a therapeutic journey through a Voice Movement Therapy process, I will trace the journey of Vicky, whom I first introduced in Volume Two of this series (Newham 1999b).

A Case Study in Five Stages of Voice Movement Therapy: Vicky

As a child, Vicky was repeatedly abused by her father who made her engage in oral sex. Her memories were very vivid, particularly the feeling of 'a numb helplessness' in her body as her father knelt on her arms to keep her down. Vicky came to work on herself through Voice Movement Therapy because, although psychotherapy had enabled her to deal with and overcome many of the issues and heal some of the damage, some problems remained. The main problem was a feeling of tightness in her throat and what she described as 'an incredibly inhibited voice'. Whenever she came to project her voice or speak up about something important, she would feel a 'stickiness' in her throat, as though her voice was 'covered with something' that made it 'dull and unable to flow fluidly'.

Stage 1: The Autobiography

During the early stages of the Voice Movement Therapy process, the client is asked to write their autobiography. Beginning with first memories and tracing their childhood through to adulthood, the client creates a written text including descriptions of their family and friends as well as major events which they feel have shaped their lives. When the task is completed, the next stage offers the client an opportunity to read the autobiography aloud – to the practitioner in individual work and to the entire ensemble in group work. The audience is asked to listen generously and not to intervene or remark in any way. The following is an excerpt from Vicky's autobiography.

Client's Autobiography: Vicky

The Girl with No Arms

My father always held my arms down and I remember them going numb and hurting. Physically it was the most painful part of the ordeal. He usually held them down with his knees, sitting on top of me, but sometimes he would clasp them with his huge hands.

He used to put his prick in my mouth and tell me to suck gently and slowly. Then he would climax and my mouth would fill up with sperm. I remember that the pain in my arms was so great that I wanted him to have an orgasm so he would release my arms. When he did I could feel the muscles in my arms tingling and it would take a while for the feeling to return to them.

After my father had left the room I would lay there for a while and then spit the sperm out into some tissues. But most of it would be swallowed. I didn't want to swallow it but it just happened so that by the time I was able to get up after he had left the room it was all in my throat.

I still have trouble with my arms today. I can't do anything for very long like writing or drawing or anything that involves the use of my arm muscles. And my throat still feels all clogged up.

The Ancient Story Circle

Often, during the reading of the autobiography, the client will express emotions provoked by particular chapters in the story. Stoic clients who tell their story with a dry detachment during therapy will, in response to reading their own writing, often weep as they speak. Also, the group of listeners will often be moved to experience a tender and vulnerable disposition as they empathise with the story told.

The exercise of writing and reading the autobiography is not only pertinent and appropriate to individual therapy; it is also a rich and enlightening process that can be conducted with many kinds of groups whose purposes may be recreational, educational or therapeutic. The process of sitting in a circle, reading your own story and listening to the stories of others acts as a kind of initiation for the members of a group who are meeting one another for the first time and who are about to embark upon a journey of discovery. The following is an excerpt from Vicky's account of the experience of reading her autobiography to the working group.

Client's Account: Vicky

Though I had told the story of my childhood sexual abuse many times in therapy – in fact with three different psychotherapists – the act of writing it as an autobiography and then reading it to an audience of others who were present with their own stories was a completely different experience.

I felt strangely separate from my story, yet at the same time completely inside it. The word that comes to mind is 'solidarity'. I felt a solidarity with the people I was reading to. I think this came from realising that I was not describing the events to an analytic therapist. I was reading my story to a group of people who were like me. I felt they were resonating with me. At times I would look up and notice others in the group crying in response to my story. Though I felt a little guilty at causing tears, at the same time I felt healed by the presence of this genuine emotion. The group seemed to be saying: 'Yes, I hear this story and I share these feelings.' Though it sounds odd, I felt loved and held.

Having a story to tell that was written on the page gave me a sense of limits. Usually, when I talk about myself, I feel like I go on and on incessantly and I never know how to finish or when to finish – as though I am looking for the right words as I speak and they never come. But having a story to tell where I had already been through the process of editing and arranging helped me deliver what I wanted to say which felt direct. I felt like I was being heard because I was getting through. I was communicating.

Stage 2: The Fairy Tale

The next stage in the Voice Movement therapy process requires the client to rewrite their autobiography as a fairy tale.

Fairy tales provide a sharp and powerful allegory for psychological experience and have been used in proliferation within therapy to help clients understand their sufferings as more than entirely personal. When a client recognises their story in the predicament of a fairy tale character, they see that what they are going through is in some ways part of a universal necessity and inevitability.

Usually, when fairy tales are used in therapy, they are employed interpretively by the therapist who draws parallels between the psychic activity within the client and the narrative and imagistic activity within the tale. But clients can be empowered greatly by transforming their own autobiographies into an original fairy tale where fathers become kings, sisters become princesses, houses become castles and the remembered environment of youth takes on legendary proportion.

European fairy tales originated in personal experience in the first instance. We may like to think of them as having descended from the magical dream time of eternity, but they have not. Fairy tales have always been grounded in social, political and psychological reality, capturing real-life events and couching them in allegory and metaphor – often in order that the tale tellers were not discovered speaking the unspeakable. In many ways, the opportunity to rewrite their autobiography as a fairy tale opens a doorway into the unspeakable aspects of the client's experience.

At this stage, the client is asked to translate their personal autobiography into a fairy tale. The client is asked to take the characters and events of the autobiography and amplify them to mythical proportion. The client is encouraged to think allegorically and to translate their personal story into a tale which carries trans-personal implications. It is often helpful for the practitioner to relate aspects of the autobiographies read by some group members to parts of well-known fairy tales, inspiring the client to make connections between the personal and the archetypal.

The following is an excerpt from the fairy tale written by Vicky.

Client's Fairytale: Vicky

The Castle of Glue

Once upon a time there was a little girl called Stuck who lived with her parents: King Tyrant and Queen Absent.

The family lived in a castle with many stairs and whenever anyone ascended or descended the stairs, the wooden boards would creak and echo throughout the castle corridors so everybody knew that someone was on the way up or on the way down.

The little girl was very unhappy because her mother was always away. She said that she had important business to do but Stuck knew that she was a Prince Chaser and that her business consisted of luring young princes into her grasp whereupon she would kiss them to death. Queen Absent loved kissing but never once kissed Stuck and this made Stuck feel very much unloved.

Because Queen Absent was away so much, King Tyrant ruled the castle and had some very strange ideas about what was good for little girls. Often, in the middle of the night or in the middle of the day, Stuck would be sitting in her parlour crying and wishing that her mother would come home and she would hear the floorboards creak as King Tyrant ascended the stairs.

She could hear the fuming and the steaming of the King's breath as her parlour door opened and the King entered carrying his kettle of glue. Stuck had seen the kettle of glue many times and hated it. In fact, just the sight of it made her bones cold.

'Now come along' the King said. 'Lay upon your bed and open your mouth as I have shown you to do'.

The little girl knew that she could not disobey the King, for his hands were like a lion's jaws and he could easily lift her from the floor and throw her onto her bed.

When Stuck was on her bed and her mouth was open the King climbed up onto the eiderdown with her, rested his knees, which were like the trunks of trees, upon her arms and poured the glue from the kettle into her mouth. Stuck wanted to cry and scream but she could not. She just lay helpless as she felt the glue trickle down into her throat.

After the King had finished the pouring he left the room and descended the stairs and Stuck knew when it was safe to move because the bottom stair had a creaking sound that was deeper than all the rest. So when she was sure that King Tyrant had reached the bottom of the stairs she would cry and try to wash away the glue with water. But by then most of it had set hard in her throat.

King Tyrant came to Stuck's parlour with a kettle of glue many times and as the years passed, Stuck's throat had so much glue in it that her voice became stuck.

Then, one day, King Tyrant was killed in an accident with his horse and at the funeral all the Kings and Queens and Princes and Princesses from all the surrounding lands said what a great man he had been. Stuck found this hard to hear because she knew that he was really a wicked man who liked to hurt children with his kettle of glue. So Stuck decided that she would tell everybody the truth about King Tyrant. However, when she opened her mouth to tell the truth, her voice would not make any sound for it was covered with so much glue. Whenever Stuck tried to tell her story, people would look at her as if she was dumb as she gurgled and babbled.

So Stuck began a journey in search of a witch or wizard, a sorcerer or a seer who could find the magic potion that would unstick her voice so that she could let everybody know the truth about King Tyrant.

Stage 3: The Journey Song

Having written and presented an autobiography, a fairy tale and a radio play, the client is now asked to write the lyrics for a song which encapsulates their life journey. The client is encouraged to combine the literal documentary writing style of the autobiography with the allegorical imagistic style of the fairytale to form a third style born from the two. This third style is written as a series of lyrics which are intended to be sung; however, the client is encouraged not to consider melody at all but to concentrate only on the literary aspects.

When the task is completed, the next stage offers the client an opportunity to read the lyrics of the journey song aloud to the practitioner, or in the case of group work to the entire ensemble. The audience is asked to listen generously and not to intervene or remark in any way.

Client's Song: Vicky

Ungluing the Voice

The following is the Journey Song which Vicky wrote and read to the therapeutic group:

Sperm and cream it makes me scream
Daddy made me suck his big Jimmy Dean
My arms went dead and the voice in my head
Told me to endure this sight obscene
I was only little with no real choice
Oh please God let me take the glue from my voice
I have tried to fight and punch and kick
To expel from my mouth his big salty prick
But the more I try the more I cry
And I choke and spew and people wonder why
For Dad is dead and no one gets
Why my voice is stuck and why I seem upset
But if I feel quite safe and no one hurts me so
I can relax my body and I start to let go
And when I do my voice unglues
And I start to hear myself afresh and anew

At the end of this rendition, Vicky recalled that after an abusive episode as she lay alone on her bed, she would often sing to herself very quietly as a way of comforting herself; it was something that no one could take from her and it gave her a place to put her distress, loneliness and shame. Now she found that reading the lyrics to her song fulfilled some of the same function. It gave her a means to release the emotions associated with her ordeal but also provided a place to put them. However, she was now eager to musicalise the lyrics and sing them; and this is the next stage in the process of Voice Movement Therapy.

Stage 4: Musicalising the Journey Song

Melody is merely exaggerated prosody, and because everybody uses prosody quite naturally, everyone has the potential ability to create melodies and make songs from their creative writing.

At this stage, the client first reads the journey song in the same way as both the autobiography and the fairy tale have been read. Then the second time, the client listens carefully to the prosody underpinning the words: where the voice rises and where it falls in pitch; where the voice sustains and where it decays; where a string of syllables or words are uttered with notes in close proximity and where the voice moves across a broad pitch scale. Then, the client voices the journey song a third time, exaggerating this prosody and allowing it to turn into the outline of a melody. The fourth time, the client sings the journey song with a tune which has arisen organically from the prosody of the reading.

Client's Account: Vicky

Changing Tune

> The tune that emerged from the prosody of my lyrics reminded me of a nursery rhyme in that it was very simple and very rhythmic. The combination between the simple, innocent child-like melody and the extremely non-innocent words put me in touch with the hideous relationship between an innocent child and sexual abuse; and it brought it home to me in a way that filled my singing with emotion. I felt like I was singing as both a child and an adult and my voice wavered between naivete and bitterness. One moment I sounded like a baby and another like an old woman.
>
> As I sang, I was reminded again that when I was little, after an abusive episode, I would often sing quietly to myself after my father had left my room. I guess this was a kind of comforting. I was maybe mothering myself. Occasionally my mother would actually sing to me. In fact this was one of the few tender things I can remember her doing. And I remember that I loved it and would not want it to stop.
>
> Singing the song created the sense of encapsulating a set of images and memories in time, as though a number of things made sense on an emotional level: my mother's singing voice, my father's abusive attacks, my loneliness as a child, my spoiled innocence and my inhibited adult voice. Now I felt I wanted to sing the song with a different quality of voice. My voice sounded restricted and weak and I felt like I wanted to get angry but did not know how.

Stage 5: The Musical Theatre Piece

The construction of a piece of Musical Theatre acts as a culmination of the previous four stages, as they did in Vicky's case.

Vicky's piece of Musical Theatre was in four scenes. Scene 1 centred around a typical domestic situation between Vicky, Vicky's mother, Vicky's father and Vicky's brother. The scene consisted of three songs linked by dialogue. At the end of Scene 1, Vicky retires to her bedroom and her mother and brother depart, leaving Vicky and her father alone in the house. Scene 2 opens with a breathtaking song sung by the father as he mounts the stairs on his way to Vicky's bedroom with the intention of abusing her. After some dialogue between Vicky and her father, he departs and Vicky sings a song of self-comfort and confusion. Scene 3 cuts to the previous generation and shows Vicky's father as a little boy in a domestic situation with his parents. This scene reveals something of the terrible upbringing which Vicky's father had. Scene 4 brings us back to the present day with Vicky as an adult in both confrontation and reconciliation with her family.

The first performance of this Musical Theatre piece was like a cross between Edgar Allen Poe and Shakespeare, revealing the dark and ominous themes of inheritance, perpetuation, perpetration and abuse. In this first rendition, all the characters had quite typical vocal qualities. The mother had a light, quiet, high pitched voice in clarinet timbre with free air in falsetto register and was portrayed as quite helpless and innocent. The father was given a loud, low pitched voice in saxophone timbre with violin, attack, disruption and in modal register and was portrayed as little more than a brute. In this initial rendition, the brother had a voice like a choir boy: high pitch, middle loudness, falsetto register and flute timbre. However, in the second rendition, everything changed. The mother and father were given identical voices: middle pitch, middle loudness, in clarinet timbre, moving between modal and falsetto with pitch fluctuation. In this rendition, the parents were portrayed as being in cahoots and allegiance, as though the mother knew what was going on and turned a blind eye and a deaf ear. The brother in this second rendition was given a voice very similar to the father's voice in the first presentation but a little less loud and with no disruption. In the third and final version, all the voices were given operatic qualities and the performance was presented as an opera with each of the characters speaking and singing with huge smiles upon their faces as they sung and spoke the scenes.

In the first rendition, all the characters wore sack cloth and, with exception of the father, had bare feet. The father meanwhile wore huge black army boots. This meant that you could not hear any of the characters move across the stage except the father, whose rhythmic stamping formed a percussive musical underpinning to the performance that was both invigorating and terrifying to watch and listen to.

In the second presentation, Vicky and her brother wore sack cloth and bare feet; but both parents wore full army uniform and wore huge black boots. They now stamped in unison and created incredible rhythmic duets with their feet as they sung together, spoke to one another and danced across the floor.

In the final rendition, all the characters wore T-shirts and trousers that were two or three sizes too small, so that the characters appeared to be bursting out of their clothes. In addition, they all accompanied their vocalising with exaggerated melodramatic gestures which were incongruent with the violence of the action. The words and actions of argumentation, abuse and conflict were juxtaposed with gestures which could have been taken from the polite etiquette of an Edwardian drawing room.

Client's Account: Vicky

To create this piece of Musical Theatre was the most empowering thing I have done. For years in therapy I had felt like the victim and product of a family structure that I could not change and that I might, if lucky, just about recover from. Then, by being asked to do this task, suddenly the whole story and all of the characters in it were at my fingertips to rearrange and restructure as I wished. Because there was an opportunity to present three different versions, it meant I was not even confined to standing by a particular interpretation – I could hold on to all of my uncertainties and contradictions.

The use of the mixture between song and dialogue was also enlightening. For years I have tried to understand what went through my father's mind as he came up those stairs time and time again. I had an idea of how he worked and how he ticked but could never express it in words or in psychological language. Yet, when asked to do this task it became apparent that I could express his perspective in song. It seemed bizarre, ludicrous and ironic to be taking such care in directing the singer to properly execute this song sung by the character who abused me throughout my childhood. Yet it was important that he did it right.

As we rehearsed the Musical Theatre piece, I had the feeling of setting the record straight, of getting things out and on show for all to see. Even though only the other members of the therapy group saw the performances, it felt that they somehow symbolised a wider audience. I was free from secrecy.

The task also encouraged me to exaggerate and recreate. I was under no pressure to get to the truth of what really happened, because I was making a piece of art. There were times during the rehearsal process that I even forgot that it was about me. At the end of the process, I realised that

I could have created ten versions, all completely different and yet all, probably, in some way true.

But most important for me was the use of the voices. Taking care to give each character definite vocal ingredients gave them a specific sharp edge and a bite of reality that connected the process with the subject matter. It was through the voice that the performers were able to emotionalise and authenticate the characters they played. There were times when the person playing my father yelled in his loud, disrupted voice that made even me shake. Also, when the voices of more than one character blended, it so perfectly symbolised the alliances formed in my family.

But what also struck me was that, although I changed the vocal ingredients for my characters for each of the three presentations, each presentation was believable. In one rendition, I gave my brother an innocent choir boy's voice to portray him as disconnected from the whole process of family emotional corruption. And indeed, I do believe that this was the nature of my brother's voice within the family. But in another rendition, I made him sound like a miniature version of my father. And, from what I know of my brother now as an adult, he has certainly taken on some of my father's less savoury features.

Because particular combinations of vocal ingredients conjured such specific images, the acoustic voices of the characters perfectly represented and communicated their social and psychological voices within the family.

I realise that some of the scenes contained quite shocking material. In the feedback session with the witnessing group, one member said that the second rendition had conjured images of Ian Brady and Myra Hindley; and many in the audience found the level of co-operation between the mother and father in the facilitating of the father's abuse unbearable and horrifying. Yet, all members of the group also said that they had felt very entertained by the productions and many of them felt guilty about that. For me this was not a problem. In fact, this was for me a central point. I suspect that my parents found the family 'goings on' very exhilarating and 'entertaining'; and I also know that they feel an enormous amount of guilt. So in many ways, the group's willingness to extract pleasure from the performance but to then question that pleasure in the light of the material was confirmation to me that I had succeeded in getting to the core of the subject.

Stage by Stage

The five stages of a therapeutic process which I have described and exemplified with the case of Vicky is just one of many routes which a client can take through the various practical methods which constitute Voice Movement Therapy. Each client and each group will necessitate a slightly different route with emphasis and weight placed on the areas most suitable to their needs. But with all stages, the therapeutic benefit seems to rest in empowering the client to diversify the acoustic voice and to use this new found malleability to embody parts of the Self which would otherwise remain mute or poorly represented. In all stages of Voice Movement Therapy, the emphasis is on creativity and artistic production rather than on analysis and reflection. Here, the stage is an arena where no part of the psyche is unworthy of placing beneath the spotlight, for all aspects of the person are considered to contain the seeds for a fresh creative enterprise.

By taking clients slowly, stage by stage, through exercises such as those explained in this book, it is amazing how quickly a client will manage the task of creating an entire musical theatre piece. I have always felt that one of the gifts which a therapist or teacher can bring to their clients is to always believe that they are capable of more than has been believed of them before.

Inside every client is a pantheon of voices and a panoply of characters waiting to burst upon the stage and make their voices heard. It is the aim of Voice Movement Therapy to provide this stage.

The Voice Movement Therapy System of Vocal Analysis

Ingredient One: Loudness

The human voice is perceived on a spectrum of loudness from quiet through moderate to loud. Loudness is determined by how hard the two vocal cords contact each other during vibration which is in turn primarily determined by the pressure of breath released from the lungs.

Increased pressure of breath expelled from the lungs draws the vocal folds together with a greater force causing them to hit each other with higher impact. Decreased air pressure, meanwhile, draws the folds together with less force, causing them to hit each other with low impact. We witness this concept when watching or listening to a pair of drawn curtains flap together during a high wind. As the pressure of the wind against the curtains increases so they flap together with greater impact, giving off a louder sound. Conversely, as the wind dies down, the curtains hit one another more gently, making the sound softer.

To increase the air pressure and therefore the loudness, we increase the contractile power of the muscles around the torso. To decrease pressure and loudness we ease off the muscular contraction.

The first vocal ingredient which we can identify in a human voice then is loudness which results from increased air pressure.

Ingredient Two: Pitch

Each vocal sound is perceived to have a certain pitch, note or fundamental tone, determined by the frequency of vocal cord vibration. This is perceived within the metaphor of high to low, though in fact does not relate to spatial dimensions but to speed of vibration in time.

The initial sound which is shaped and coloured to produce a unique human voice is made by the vibration of the vocal cords. These two folds of tissue, also known as the vocal folds, lay stretched out in the larynx. At the front they are attached to the

Adam's apple or thyroid cartilage and at the back they are connected to two movable cartilages called the arytenoids.

These two pieces of tissue are further attached to the trachea and the surrounding inner walls of the larynx by a complex set of muscles known collectively as the intrinsic laryngeal musculature. During normal breathing the vocal folds lay at rest, one each side of the larynx, like an open pair of curtains allowing air to pass freely through a window. The hole between the vocal folds through which air passes is called the glottis. However, adjustments in the distribution of tension in the laryngeal musculature can cause the vocal folds to close, preventing air from entering or leaving the trachea, like a thick pair of curtains drawn tightly shut across a window.

The sound of the human voice is generated by the rapid and successive opening and closure of the vocal cords many times per second and it is to this process that people refer when they speak of the vibration of the vocal cords. This rapid vibration of the vocal cords causes the expelled air from the lungs to be released through the glottis in a series of infinitesimal puffs which create a sound wave.

The faster the vocal cords vibrate the higher the pitch. The slower they vibrate, the lower the pitch. As a useful point of reference, to sing middle C the vocal cords must vibrate about 256 times per second. To sing the A above middle C they must vibrate at around 440 times per second.

Because the vocal folds are attached front and back to the thyroid and arytenoid cartilages, which are in turn connected to muscle tissue, they can be stretched out by tensile adjustment in the laryngeal musculature making them longer, thinner and more tense. When this happens, like all elastic objects which are tightened, they vibrate at a higher frequency which produces a higher sound or pitch. Conversely, an alternative adjustment of the laryngeal musculature causes the vocal folds to slacken, so that they become shorter, thicker and more lax. When this happens, like all elastic objects which are relaxed, they vibrate at a lower frequency and the consequent sound of the voice deepens in pitch.

In establishing a component system of intuitive vocal analysis, the second physiologically generated ingredient of perceivable acoustic sound which we can identify as being present in a person's voice is therefore the pitch, also referred to as the note or the tone.

Ingredient Three: Pitch Fluctuation

The pitch of the voice sustains more or less constancy or fluctuation in a given time. This is determined by the shifting frequencies of vocal cord vibration.

During vibration, the vocal cords may not remain absolutely constant in their speed of vibration over a given time and consequently they may produce a pitch fluctuation.

There are two components to this pitch fluctuation: interval distance and time. Interval distance is the magnitude of the pitch fluctuation. For example, a voice which fluctuates from a vibrational frequency of 440 to 450 times per second makes a pitch fluctuation across a tiny interval from the A above middle C on a piano to a sound not even high enough to sound the A-sharp above it. A voice meanwhile which fluctuates from 440 to 493 times per second makes a pitch fluctuation across a large interval equivalent to going from the A above middle C on the piano to the B above it. The term interval thereby denotes the magnitude of the frequency jump between two specific notes or pitches.

The next factor, time, is the speed with which the fluctuations are made. A very slow alternation between 440 times per second, which is the A above middle C on the piano and 450 times per second, which does not have a note on the piano, may well sound 'out of tune' to a listener. But if the same inconsistency is quickened it may sound like a very professional singing voice. Indeed, very fast fluctuations in vocal cord vibration over a very small pitch interval constitutes what is known as vibrato, that deliberate flutter which is heard in the classical European voice. If a singer produces such pitch fluctuations too slowly, or takes them across too great a pitch interval, the skill of the vibrato turns into what we hear as untuneful singing.

The third vocal ingredient which we can identify within the human voice then is pitch fluctuation which under certain conditions would be referred to as vibrato and under others may be called inconsistency or untunefulness. However, what is heard as pleasant and unpleasant, as an acceptable interval and an unacceptable interval is culturally determined.

Ingredient Four: Register

The voice is produced with what is perceived as a certain register, either modal, falsetto, whistle or vocal fry. The voice can also be perceived as being composed of a blended combination of modal and falsetto.

If a person begins to sing the lowest note possible and rises one note at a time up to the highest he or she can sing, it will be possible to discern alterations in the timbre at certain points, as though the person has 'changed voices'. Amongst the changes which a listener would observe would be a shift of 'register'.

Most voices have two main registers in singing, known as modal and falsetto. The most familiar and easily recognisable changes between the modal and falsetto registers occurs when a man or a woman ascends upwards from a deep pitch towards higher ones during which at a certain point a 'register break' occurs where the voice 'breaks' out of modal and into falsetto. It is this register break which is exaggerated and musicalised in the yodelling style of singing originating in Switzerland. In classical European singing, singers learn to blend the two registers together so that the break is not heard.

Scientific instrumentational investigation has not yet been able to explain exactly what does cause the audible shifts in timbre which give rise to particular registers. We do know, however, that the alterations in the size of the glottis are instrumental in effecting change in what is known as voice register.

Both modal and falsetto register can be produced on low and high pitches, though the higher the voice in pitch the more natural and easier it is to produce falsetto and the lower the pitch of the voice the more natural and easier it is produce modal. In addition, through precise control of the laryngeal musculature, a vocal sound can be produced which blends together the two registers into a single quality.

If the vocal folds remain closed along the majority of their length so that only a minimal portion is vibrating, making a tiny glottis, the voice quality produced is like a piercing scream and is known as the whistle register. Because this requires extreme tension in the vocal folds, the pitch of the whistle register is always very high. If, in contradistinction, the vocal folds are very lax and their entire length is vibrating then the quality of voice often produced is like a low, airy grumble known as the vocal fry register which, due to the lack of tension in the folds, is always produced on low notes.

The fourth ingredient to vocal sound which we can therefore identify is vocal register, of which the two main ones are modal and falsetto with two less frequently heard registers named whistle and vocal fry.

Ingredient Five: Harmonic Timbre – Flute, Clarinet, Saxophone

Harmonic timbre is the particular quality of the voice determined by the shape and dimensions of the vocal tract or voice tube. Harmonic timbre may be arbitrarily divided into three qualities arising from a short, narrow tract, a medium length and diameter tract and a fully lengthened and dilated tract. These are given the names flute, clarinet and saxophone respectively.

The vocal tract which runs upwards from the larynx, becomes the pharynx, turns into the oro-pharynx and curls round to become the mouth is capable of altering its size and shape. And it is the shape and movement of this tube which governs so much of the specific quality of a voice which we hear, regardless of the degree and combination of other vocal ingredients.

To understand how the movement and configuration of this tube affects vocal quality it will be useful to imagine three crude tubes, closed at the bottom but open at the top, all made of exactly the same substance but constructed to different diameters and different lengths. The first is short and narrow; the second is relatively longer and wider; and the third is much longer and more dilated again. Imagine that we hold a tuning fork which produces middle C over the top of each tube in turn and listen to the sound of the note echoing or resonating inside the tubes. In moving from listening to the sound inside the first tube to the same note echoing or resonating in the second and then the third, the listener would hear a change of timbre. Probably, the first tube would sound more comparable to a flute, the second tube would sound more comparable to the clarinet, whilst the sound produced by the third tube would sound more akin to the saxophone; they would all however sound the note C.

With regard to voice production, both the length and the diameter of the voice tube or vocal tract can alter, producing a variety of timbres, yet the pitch can be held constant by an unchanging frequency of vocal cord vibration. So, imagine that instead of a tuning fork at the top of three crude tubes, you have vibrating vocal cords at the bottom of one tube which can change its length and diameter to assume the relative dimensions of all three tubes. This gives some idea of how different timbres are created by the vocal instrument.

The vocal tract which runs downwards from the lips to the larynx is an elastic tube which can assume various lengths and diameters.

In place of the three crude tubes, we can now therefore pinpoint three arbitrary degrees of dilation and lengthening along the path of the vocal tract. The first compares to a flute-like tube, whereby the larynx is high in the neck and the tract is quite constricted creating a short, narrow tube, such as when we blow a kiss or whistle. The second configuration, which compares to the clarinet-like tube, is characterised by a lower position of the larynx in the neck creating a longer tube which is more dilated, such as when we steam up a pair of glasses. The third configuration, which compares to the saxophone-like tube, is characterised by a complete descent of the larynx in the neck, creating a long tube with maximum dilation, such as when we yawn.

If the vibratory frequency of the vocal cords is maintained at a constant, say at 256 times per second, producing middle C, whilst the vocal tract moves from flute configuration through clarinet configuration to saxophone configuration, the effect will be to sing the same note with three very distinct timbres, comparable to that achieved when playing the note C on a tuning fork held above the three separate crude tubes imagined earlier.

In Voice Movement Therapy, we give the vocal timbre produced by a short, narrow voice tube the instrumental name flute timbre; we name the vocal timbre produced by a medium length and diameter tube clarinet timbre; and we call the vocal timbre produced by a fully lengthened and dilated voice tube saxophone timbre.

Ingredient Six: Nasality

The human voice may be heard as possessing a spectral degree of nasal resonance from none through moderate to high. When nasal resonance is severely inhibited or blocked, the sound may metaphorically be described as lacking in violin; when nasal resonance is full, the voice may be described as possessing a high degree of violin.

Some of the sound wave created by the vibrating vocal cords may pass through the nasal passages which runs from the oro-pharynx up above the roof of the mouth and out through the nose and the amount of air which passes through this tract influences the vocal quality. The passage of air through the nasal tube can be controlled by the raising and lowering of the soft palate which closes and opens the port of entry to the nasal tract respectively. At one extreme, the movement of air through this passage can be completely prevented and at the other, the maximum amount of air capable of passing through this port can travel through the nasal passages and out of the nose. Between these two extremes, an entire spectrum of nasal air flow is possible.

When the soft palate is lowered allowing maximum nasal resonance, the voice is described as possessing a lot of violin. When the soft palate is closed so that nasal resonance is inhibited, the voice is described as lacking in violin.

The sixth ingredient of the human voice which we can identify is therefore the degree of nasal resonance which is given the instrumental and metaphorical name of violin and perceived on a spectrum from none through moderate to high.

Ingredient Seven: Free Air

The quality of the voice is perceived as being more or less breathy or airy, perceived on a spectrum from none through moderate to high and determined by the volume or quantity of air flowing through the glottis.

Although the vocal cords are opening and closing very quickly, they may not push tightly together when they close. If the vocal cords are closed, but are not kept pushed together tightly, then even during their closed phase, air can pass through the folds in the form of a trickle or a seepage. When this happens the voice has a certain breathiness which is described as a voice rich in free air. A voice may also be rich in free air if the glottis is enlarged during vocal cord vibration.

The seventh ingredient of the voice is therefore free air which is perceived on a spectrum from little through moderate to high.

Ingredient Eight: Attack

The voice is perceived as having greater or lesser attack, determined by the impact under which the vocal folds come together during phonation.

Unlike curtains, the vocal cords are not only reliant upon the wind from the lungs for their movement as they are connected to muscles which are fed by nerves. It is therefore possible to vary the impact of vocal cord contact without major changes in air pressure, increasing and decreasing vocal cord impact, creating sounds with varying degrees of glottal attack whilst maintaining a constant loudness.

The eighth ingredient of vocal sound which we can identify is therefore glottal attack, determined by the impact of vocal fold contact.

Ingredient Nine: Disruption

The human voice may or may not be to some degree disrupted, that is broken or sporadically interrupted in a way which appears to interfere with the continuity of the tone. This can be caused by friction or uneven contact between the vocal folds, by other tissue structures coming into contact with the vocal cords during vibration or it can be caused by intermittent silence breaking up the tone.

We have so far assumed that during vocalisation the vocal folds are drawn together so as to meet flush and smooth along their vibrating edge, preventing air from escaping other than during their rhythmic opening and thereby producing a clear tone. However, under certain circumstances, not only may the vocal folds not meet under enough pressure to prevent air escaping, but the vocal folds may crash together unevenly, their edges being corrugated and uneven, rubbing against each other and producing a sound which sounds broken, frictional, rough and discontinuous. These broken sounds are referred to as disrupted.

At other times, such as during laryngitis or influenza or when the vocal cords are damaged, the vocal tone may be intermittently broken with silences. In addition, other tissue structures in the larynx may come into contact with the vocal cords during vocalisation, interrupting the tone.

The ninth vocal ingredient which we can identify is therefore disruption.

Ingredient Ten: Articulation

The human voice may be perceived as producing sounds which appear close to a sound usable within the spoken language of a particular culture and which are produced by the shapes of the vocal tract in combination with the movements of tongue and lips.

It is the harmonic embellishment of a pitch caused by changing dimensions of the vocal tract that gives rise to specific timbres which we call vowels and which are born from very specific shapes of the vocal tract.

In addition, the air flow from the larynx may be momentarily stopped. Sometimes the air is stopped at the back of the mouth, such as 'k'. Other consonants are produced by interrupting the air flow at the lips, such as 'p' or 'b'. Some articulate sounds are used in one language but not in another. For example, 'ach' is used in German and Arabic but not in English.

The tenth and last vocal ingredient is therefore articulation, composed of vowels and consonants.

The System of Ten Vocal Ingredients

From a simple understanding of vocal physiology it is therefore possible to deduce ten ingredients which combine to form the sound of the human voice. When listening to a person vocalising, whether in song, or in speech, whether in a therapeutic or a creative context, a practitioner can be trained to listen to the voice in terms of these ingredients which provide the basis for interpretation, analysis and training. These ingredients of vocal expression form the core of a system of Voicework which is both an analytic profile for interpreting voices, a psycho-therapeutic means by which to investigate the way psychological material is communicated through specific vocal qualities, a training system for developing the expressivity of voices and a physiotherapeutic means by which to release the voice from functional misuse.

I have presented extensive recordings of the ten vocal ingredients with a detailed explanation of the Voice Movement Therapy system of vocal analysis on a set of audio tapes *The Singing Cure: Liberating Self Expression Through Voice Movement Therapy* (Newham 1998).

To recap, here are the ten ingredients.

Ingredient One: Loudness
The human voice is perceived on a spectrum of loudness from quiet through moderate to loud. Loudness is determined by how hard the two vocal cords contact each other during vibration which is in turn primarily determined by the pressure of breath released from the lungs.

Ingredient Two: Pitch
Each vocal sound is perceived to have a certain pitch, note or fundamental tone, determined by the frequency of vocal cord vibration. This is perceived within the metaphor of high to low, though in fact does not relate to spatial dimensions but to speed of vibration in time.

Ingredient Three: Pitch Fluctuation

The pitch of the voice sustains more or less constancy or fluctuation in a given time. This is determined by the shifting frequencies of vocal cord vibration.

Ingredient Four: Register

The voice is produced with what is perceived as a certain register, either modal, falsetto, whistle or vocal fry. The voice can also be perceived as being composed of a blended combination of modal and falsetto.

Ingredient Five: Harmonic Timbre – Flute, Clarinet, Saxophone

Harmonic timbre is the particular quality of the voice determined by the shape and dimensions of the vocal tract or voice tube. Harmonic timbre may be arbitrarily divided into three qualities arising from a short, narrow tract, a medium length and diameter tract and a fully lengthened and dilated tract. These are given the names flute, clarinet and saxophone respectively.

Ingredient Six: Nasality

The human voice may be heard as possessing a spectral degree of nasal resonance from none through moderate to high. When nasal resonance is severely inhibited or blocked, the sound may metaphorically be described as lacking in violin; when nasal resonance is full, the voice may be described as possessing a high degree of violin.

Ingredient Seven: Free Air

The quality of the voice is perceived as being more or less breathy or airy, perceived on a spectrum from none through moderate to high and determined by the volume or quantity of air flowing through the glottis.

Ingredient Eight: Attack

The voice is perceived as having greater or lesser attack, determined by the impact under which the vocal folds come together during phonation.

Ingredient Nine: Disruption

The human voice may or may not be to some degree disrupted, that is broken or sporadically interrupted in a way which appears to interfere with the continuity of the tone. This can be caused by friction or uneven contact between the vocal folds, by other tissue structures coming into contact with the vocal cords during vibration or it can be caused by intermittent silence breaking up the tone.

Ingredient Ten: Articulation

The human voice may be perceived as producing sounds which appear close to a sound usable within the spoken language of a particular culture and which are produced by the shapes of the vocal tract in combination with the movements of tongue and lips.

Further Information

For further information including a list of qualified Voice Movement Therapy practitioners, a full prospectus of training and courses and a complete list of currently available resources including the accompanying video and set of audio tapes, please contact:

The Administrator
Voice Movement Therapy
PO Box 4218
London
SE22 0JE
Tel: (+44) (0) 181 693 9502
Fax: (+44) (0) 181 299 6127
Email: info@voicework.com

Information can also be accessed on the Voice Movement Therapy Web site: www.voicework.com

References

Fordham, M. (1985) 'Explorations into the Self.' *Library of Analytical Psychology*, Volume 7. London: Academic Press.

Hillman, J. (1977) *Re-Visioning Psychology*. New York: Harper & Row.

Jung, C.G. (1953) *The Collected Works of C G Jung*, Bollingen Series XX, edited by H. Read, M. Fordham, G. Adler and W. McGuire. Princeton, New Jersey: Princeton University Press and London: Routledge and Kegan Paul.

Jung, C.G. (1968) *C G Jung and Herman Hesse: A Record Of Two Friendships*, Miguel Serrano, translated by F. MacShane, New York: Schocken.

Newham, P. (1997a) *Shouting for Jericho: The Work of Paul Newham on the Human Voice*. Video. London: Tigers Eye/Class Productions.

Newham, P. (1997b) *Therapeutic Voicework: Principles and Practice for the Use of Singing as a Therapy*. London: Jessica Kingsley Publishers.

Newham, P. (1997c) *The Prophet of Song: The Life and Work of Alfred Wolfsohn*. London: Tigers Eye.

Newham. P. (1998) *The Singing Cure: Liberating Self Expression Through Voice Movement Therapy*. Audio cassettes. Boulder, Colorado: Sounds True.

Newham, P. (1999a) *Using Voice and Movement in Therapy: The Practical Application of Voice Movement Therapy*. London: Jessica Kingsley Publishers.

Newham, P. (1999b) *Using Voice and Song in Therapy: The Practical Application of Voice Movement Therapy*. London: Jessica Kingsley Publishers.

Redfearn, J. (1985) 'My Self, My Many Selves.' *Library of Analytical Psychology*, Volume 6. London: Academic Press.

Index

.